Biomedical Ethics Reviews • 1987

T0320717

Biomedical Ethics Reviews

Edited by

James M. Humber and Robert F. Almeder

Board of Editors

William Bechtel
Department of Philosophy
Georgia State University
Atlanta, Georgia

Thomas H. Murray
University of Texas Medical Branch
Galveston, Texas

William J. Curran
Harvard School of Public Health
Boston, Massachusetts

James Muyskens
Hunter College
New York, New York

Kurt Hirschhorn
The Mount Sinai Medical Center
New York, New York

James Rachels
University of Alabama
Birmingham, Alabama

Richard Hull
State Univ. of New York, Buffalo
Amherst, New York

Richard Wasserstrom
University of California
Santa Cruz, California

Biomedical Ethics Reviews • 1987

Edited by

JAMES M. HUMBER
and ROBERT F. ALMEDER

Georgia State University, Atlanta, Georgia

Humana Press • Clifton, New Jersey

Copyright © 1988 by The Humana Press Inc.
Crescent Manor
PO Box 2148
Clifton, NJ 07015 USA

All rights in any form whatsoever reserved.

No part of this book may be reproduced, stored in a retrieval system, or trans-
mitted in any form or by any means (electronic, mechanical, photocopying, micro-
filming, recording, or otherwise) without written permission from the publisher.

Printed in the United States of America.

The Library of Congress has cataloged this serial title as follows:

Biomedical ethics reviews—1983-   Clifton, NJ: Humana Press, c1982-

v.; 25 cm—(Contemporary issues in biomedicine, ethics, and society)
Annual.
Editors: James M. Humber and Robert F. Almeder.
ISSN 0742–1796 = Biomedical ethics reviews.

1. Medical ethics—Periodicals. I. Humber, James M.   II. Almeder, Robert F.
III. Series.

[DNLM: 1. Ethics, Medical—periodicals. W1 B615 (P)]

R724.B493   174'.2'05—dc19   84-640015
                                                          AACR 2   MARC-S

Contents

The Nurse's Role
Rights and Responsibilities

Preface

Biomedical Ethics Reviews • 1987 is the fifth volume in
a series of texts designed to review and update the literature
on issues of central importance in bioethics today. Three
topics are discussed in the present volume: (1) Prescribing
Drugs for the Aged and Dying; (2) Animals as a Source of
Human Transplant Organs, and (3) The Nurse's Role: Rights
and Responsibilities. Each topic constitutes a separate section in our text; introductory essays briefly summarize the
contents of each section.

Bioethics is, by its nature, interdisciplinary in character.
Recognizing this fact, the authors represented in the present
volume have made every effort to minimize the use of technical jargon. At the same time, we believe the purpose of providing a review of the recent literature, as well as of advancing
bioethical discussion, is admirably served by the pieces col-
lected herein. We look forward to the next volume in our
series, and very much hope the reader will also.

James M. Humber
Robert F. Almeder

Contributors

Sarah Bachrach • *Department of Philosophy, University of Western Ontario, London, Ontario, Canada*

Marsha D. M. Fowler • *Consulting Ethicist, Pasadena, California*

R. G. Frey • *Department of Philosophy, Bowling Green State University, Bowling Green, Ohio*

Barry Hoffmaster • *Department of Philosophy, University of Western Ontario, London, Ontario, Canada*

Darlene Aulds Martin • *School of Nursing, University of Texas, Austin, Texas*

James L. Nelson • *Department of Philosophy, St. John's University, Collegeville, Minnesota*

Richard Werner • *Department of Philosophy, Hamilton College, Clinton, New York*

Ron Yezzi • *Department of Philosophy, Mankato State University, Mankato, Minnesota*

Prescribing Drugs for the Aged and Dying

Introduction

In their essay, "Ethical Issues in Prescribing Drugs for the Aged and the Dying," Barry Hoffmaster and Sarah Bachrach seek to specify the conditions under which the elderly and the dying lose their decision-making responsibilities in matters affecting their own health. When do the elderly and the dying lose their autonomy in determining what is in their best interest? When in fact are the aged and the dying harmed by the inadvertence and ignorance of their health-care providers, poor communication between them and their providers, and the unwillingness of society to fund adequately health care for them? Moreover, one major problem for both patients and providers is distinguishing the effects of the normal phenomenon of aging from the effects of disease. Ignorance in this latter area could lead to the acceptance of problems that could be treated and the prescribing of medications that are inappropriate or harmful. Altogether too frequently, vital decisions affecting the health of the elderly are made by others when the elderly are more than competent to make such decisions.

Hoffmaster and Bachrach describe the various questionable ways in which health-providers succeed in harming their patients. In the conclusion the authors describe what they take to be the main moral problem in providing health care to the elderly. The problem is that individuals who have been responsible for themselves and their families for most of their lives are disenfranchised by age, regardless of whether doing so is warranted by infirmity. They move from being responsible to being an obligation. Hence their lives are controlled by others and open to others. The problems that arise with respect to prescribing medications flow, in large measure, from this general attitude toward the elderly.

In the second essay in this section, "Prescribing Drugs for the Aged and Dying," Ron Yezzi lays down guidlines for prescribing drugs to the aged and the elderly. These guidelines emerge after a consideration of various pointed cases, legal and ethical principles, the types of drugs available for treatment of the elderly and the dying, and the ethical decisions involved in prescribing drugs.

Some of the major questions confronted in this essay are: When, if at all, is it *ethically* acceptable for a physician to administer a lethal injection in accordance with a patient's wishes, when the patient is mentally competent, has maintained the same wish for several years, and is suffering from a severely debilitating terminal disease? When, if at all, is it ethically acceptable to administer a lethal injection (or withhold ordinary treatment) in the absence of a patient's wishes, when the patient is mentally incompetent, and is suffering from a severely debilitating terminal disease? Should we ever honor a patient's request to refuse standard treatment for an otherwise fatal disease when the request is coupled with a demand for treatment regarded as worthless by the medical community? Should physicians acquiesce in a competent patient's request to actively direct his own drug treatment for pain relief? And finally, to what extent should narcotics be used for pain control when the side effects may hasten the moment of death? In seeking to answer such questions, the author lists five basic ethical principles that should be acceptable to all health care providers. Thereafter, guidelines for answering the above questions and treating specific cases are derived from the acceptable moral principles in a way that allows us to resolve ethical problems in specific cases.

Ethical Issues
in Prescribing Drugs
for the Aged and the Dying

Barry Hoffmaster and Sarah Bachrach

Introduction

There are two competing conceptions of the nature of biomedical ethics. One, the Platonic conception, holds that morality is a body of theoretical knowledge obtained through reason and that practical ethics consists of applying this knowledge—a moral theory or a set of moral principles—to cases. The facts of a case are subsumed under the theory or set of principles to yield a determinate conclusion about the course of action that ought to be adopted. The other, the Aristotelian conception, holds that morality is the outcome of reason, common sense, and experience operating in the realm of concrete moral problems. Morality is essentially a pragmatic, not a speculative, activity, so there is no appreciable gulf between theoretical knowledge and its application to practical affairs. Morality involves identifying and appraising the values that conflict in a case, then searching for strategies that either will remove or resolve the conflict. To the extent that moral knowledge exists, it comprises the lessons that can be drawn from this analysis and comparison of cases.

The Aristotelian view of morality as an intrinsically practical enterprise provides a better understanding of the ethical issues that arise in prescribing drugs for the aged and dying. To be sure, a central question in biomedical ethics—when, if ever, health care providers can arrogate to themselves the right to make decisions on behalf of patients—also arises with respect to the elderly and dying. With this group, though, the question acquires a different cast for two reasons. First, decision-making authority, even for competent elderly persons, is routinely relegated to others, notably the family. Middle-aged children assume responsibility for their elderly parents as a matter of course. At breakfast in a restaurant, for example, a middle-aged son intercedes to repeat in a louder voice the order of his elderly but clearly competent and alert father. He does so unthinkingly, without giving his father the opportunity to repeat his order to the waitress. The assumption that elderly people need help dealing with the world is unconscious and pervasive. This attitude undoubtedly has many causes, but it may in part reflect the inability of both parties to transform the parent–child relationship into an adult–adult relationship. In any event the elderly and dying are treated differently from other adults in that the presumption frequently is against their exercise of decision-making responsiblility. Second, elderly patients can be easily coerced. The threat of placement in a nursing home if they do not "go along" or comply with a recommendation hangs ominously over the heads of many elderly patients. The presumption against the elderly and dying participating in decisions concerning their own care should not exist; nor should their vulnerability be exploited.

The prevailing goal here, as elsewhere in health care, is uncontroversial—above all, do no harm. But here, perhaps even more so than in other areas of health care, the notion of harm must be understood expansively. Harm includes violations of a person's dignity as well as violations of a person's physical and psychological integrity. Illness for the elderly can be debilitating of spirit as well as body. One of the main moral challenges associated with managing the health problems of elderly persons is to allow them to retain their dignity and their sense of what is fitting and proper. That can be accomplished by allowing them to participate in decisions and thereby retain control over their lives. Control also contributes to healthy aging. The physical impact of growing old can be managed because changes occur gradually, giving a person time to adapt and deal with accompanying stress. Adaptation, however, presupposes the ability to control one's response to change, and control, in turn, presupposes choice.

There are, of course, situations in which the view of the family or medical team will have to prevail, but those situations should remain the exception, not the rule. The presumption should be in favor of, rather than against, decision-making responsibility by elderly and dying patients. Most important, when this responsibility is removed, the sense of a greater tragedy should not be lost. The tragedy is greater because the realm in which choice can be exercised progressively narrows with age. Death takes away one's spouse and one's friends. Disease takes away one's health and independence. Society takes away one's esteem and respect. As the number of choices wanes, the significance of each waxes. That lesson is as important in medical care as it is anywhere else.

The pressing problem that remains, though, is determining when a situation is truly an exception to the presumption in favor of elderly and dying patients exercising decision-making responsibility. In what circumstances can this presumption be rebutted? Balancing, in a concrete case, the value of exercising autonomy against the value of promoting what is perceived by another to be in the patient's best interest cannot be done by appealing to a general philosophical theory or a set of general moral principles. Instead, the relevant factors of individual cases must be identified and assessed, and judgment must be exercised in counterpoising the factors to arrive at a decision. The point of the Aristotelian conception of morality is that such judgment requires common sense, experience, and reason, not merely facility at abstract thinking.

Another pressing problem is to recognize the ways in which aged and dying patients are harmed, largely as a result of the inadvertence and ignorance of their health care providers, poor communication between them and their providers, and the unwillingness of society to fund health care for this group of patients adequately. A major problem for both patients and their providers is distinguishing the effects of the normal phenomena of aging from the effects of diseases. Ignorance in this regard can lead to the acceptance of problems that could be treated and the prescribing of medications that are inappropriate. It is these more practical concerns, discovered through experience and remedied by education, common sense, and commitment, that dominate in the care of the aged and dying. The ethical problems in this area do not provide much grist for the philosophic mill, but they do provide considerable grist for the biomedical ethics and political mills.

The Geriatric Population

The rapid expansion of the elderly population in the United States and Canada is a major worry for health care planners. The number of persons over 65 years of age is predicted to double by 2030, with the fastest growing segment of this group being persons over 85 years of age. By the year 2000 25% of the population in the United States will be at least 65 years old.[1] People are living longer because of advances in medical technology and the adoption of healthier lifestyles. Physicians, hospitals, insurance companies, and society are concerned about the costs of caring for an expanding population that is both medically fragile and medically sophisticated. Blue Cross/Blue Shield insurance is expensive and covers only hospital care; it does not pay for outpatient office visits or for drugs. Health Maintenance Organizations (HMOs), which cover office visits and hospital care but not the cost of medication, are just beginning to enroll the elderly. They cater to young, working people who do not have chronic diseases and who use medical services sparingly. HMOs that do accept older persons are taking healthy 65-year-olds rather than medically fragile 80-year-olds.

Medicare and Medicaid pay for the health care of the majority of elderly persons. Medicare, which is entitlement insurance based on work history, covers hospital admissions and physician visits. Only Medicare B, a private insurance plan that can be purchased by those on Medicare, pays for medications. Eligibility for Medicaid, which covers office visits, medications, and hospital admissions (if the client does not have Medicare), is based upon income. Many elderly persons who reside in nursing homes end up relying on Medicaid to cover their room and board as well.

In one study a group of nursing home patients was found to have an average of six diagnoses of medical problems and to be on an average of twelve medications for the management of these problems.[2] If the costs of the drugs typically prescribed for a patient with hypertension and arthritis, just two common maladies of the aged, were calculated, the total per month would be $138 ($30 for a diuretic taken once a day, $48 for a long-acting beta blocker taken once a day, and $60 for an anti-inflammatory taken four times a day). Most people, when they retire at 65 or 70, are forced to live off savings and pensions, or to be supported by their families or Medicaid. At the same time as their incomes are diminishing, they are experiencing more medical problems and increasingly expensive health care needs. Thus cost becomes a major ethical consideration in prescribing drugs for the aged. If elderly patients cannot afford to have prescriptions filled, they may be deterred from consulting their health care providers, with the consequence that medical problems might be undetected or exacerbated. The link between inadequate income and medical harm is short, direct, and mutually reinforcing. It is well known that poverty and medical problems are associated. The more impoverished a person is, the more medical problems he or she is likely to have. And as the number of medical problems increases, so does the difficulty of paying for the medications to manage those problems.

Problems for Aged Patients

The Locus of Decision Making

A general problem of growing old in North America is the loss of esteem that accompanies the loss of a salary. Esteem fades when one retires and no longer is contributing productively to society. Diminishing esteem can be manifested in declining respect for an elderly person's decision-making capacity. The right to make decisions is a central issue in both medical ethics and medical jurisprudence, but the issue becomes particularly acute for the aged, when decision-making authority seems to be transferred, willingly or unwillingly on both sides, to the family. Relatives not uncommonly "drag" elderly patients to the medical provider and insist that they take their medications. These relatives may be supportive, caring, and well intentioned, but they may also be ignoring or overriding the wishes of elderly persons and thereby compromising their dignity.

The following case illustrates the general conflict that can exist between patient and family.

> Ms. B, who is 78 years old, lives by herself in the house where she raised her family and has resided for the past 40 years. She has been coping well with several chronic diseases, but recently slipped on the floor and fractured her hip. During her hospitalization her family decided that her house is too big. They are concerned that she will have a heart attack and be unattended for days before help arrives. The family has discussed the situation with their mother's social worker and medical provider, and they have collectively decided that nursing home placement is necessary. When the issue is raised with Ms. B, she cries and refuses to give up her home. A

"compromise" that will require Ms. B to live in a
nursing home for "a few months" while she is recu-
perating finally is reached.

This, unfortunately, is a typical scenario. Sometimes the reason
for placement is less laudable, for instance, the family is embar-
rassed by the cluttered, dirty, or squalid conditions in which their
mother lives. In any event the family has no intention of allowing
their mother to go home and so clears out her house. The mother
is tearful in the nursing home. She repeatedly asks when she will
return home, but as the months go by the discussions become
progressively less frequent, or an acute illness, such as pneumonia
or bed sores, occurs, which "confirms" the wisdom of the placement. One never will know whether depression has made a patient
more susceptible to infection, or whether the patient might have had
years of uneventful, healthy living had she returned home.

When the elderly relative resides with the family, the decision
can be even more difficult. For example, an 84-year-old father,
who lives with his daughter and son-in-law, falls periodically
because he has poor balance. At night the risk of harm is even greater because he sleepwalks and sometimes falls during his somnabu-
listic journeys. In addition, he has a urinary problem that requires
him to get up frequently to go to the bathroom, which is at the top
of the stairs. His family resists putting him in a nursing home, but,
needless to say, does not sleep well. It might be only a matter of
time until the limits of the family's ability to cope are reached.

Both family members and professionals make decisions to place
persons in nursing homes with the best intentions and with enorm-
ous guilt, but the decisions are made on behalf of the elderly, not by
the elderly. The only real solution is creative thinking and funding
that will provide the resources to alleviate such difficult situations
or at least make them tolerable. The availability of electronic
devices that allow a conscious person to signal when he or she has
fallen and other emergency alert systems is one example. The

practice of postal workers checking on elderly persons when they deliver mail and the development of "granny homes," portable living units that can be rented and erected in a back yard, are other examples. Without such creative problem solving, forced placement in a nursing home remains an inevitable prospect for many elderly persons.

Forced placement, whether it is a matter of necessity or more a matter of convenience, has clear implications for prescribing medications. Soon after individuals are unwillingly placed in nursing homes, their medical providers usually receive a call from the nursing staff, reporting that they are not "settling in." The person might be constantly pacing and crying, for example, so the nursing staff requests that a sedative be ordered. The sedation probably will continue for six to eight weeks, until the person has been "institutionalized," but because of the person's mental state, the decision about taking a sedative never will be put to him or her.

The next case shows how the responsibility to decide what drugs one will take can be explicitly removed from an elderly patient.

> Ms. P, who is 74 years old and has arthritis as her major diagnosis, complains to her health care provider that neither aspirin nor Motrin is controlling her pain. The provider discusses with her the side effects of stronger medications, which include drowsiness and confusion. Ms. P assures her provider that she has never abused drugs and that she would take the stronger medications only when absolutely necessary. The provider nevertheless defers Ms. P's request and subsequently discusses the side effects of stronger medications with Ms. P's family. Because they are worried about dangerous side effects more than Ms. P's pain, they decide to give Ms. P a different medication, but one that is no stronger. The provider tells Ms. P that this new drug (Naproxen) works a little differently from those she

has been taking, but is much stronger and should
control her pain.

The medical provider and family have secretly overruled Ms. P's
decision about the medication she requires for effective pain control and deceived her. Their decision may be well intentioned, and
the new drug may in fact relieve Ms. P's pain, but neither justifies
the disrespect and manipulation that have occurred. This course of
action seems wrong in itself. In addition, the desired good consequences might not materialize. It is possible that Ms. P will never
discover the subterfuge, but conspiracies can create guilt and
unease that are difficult to conceal. If Ms. P senses this discomfort,
she could have misgivings that would lead her to not fill the
prescription or not take the new drug. Ms. P might decide to suffer
to prove that she does not abuse drugs, or she might fortuitously
learn that Naproxen is no stronger than what she has been taking
and double or triple her dose. Both outcomes would be bad for Ms.
P's health, and the ensuing mistrust could damage her relationship
with her provider. Medical providers and families need to recognize the value of having elderly persons assume responsibility for
their care, as well as their own limitations in deciding what is in the
best interest of another person.

Prescribing for Behavior Control

The issue of nonparticipation in decision making becomes particularly dramatic when a drug is prescribed to control behavior.

Ms. F, who is 83 years old, is at best forgetful and
at worst senile. She comes to the nurses' station at
10:00 a.m. to ask if her daughter, who visits after
work at 5:00 p.m., has arrived. When told the time,
Ms. F returns to her room. Within ten minutes she
is back at the nurses' station with the same question.

Her trips to the nurses' station occur at frequent
intervals throughout the day and have become so
disruptive that the nurses have lost sympathy for her
and just want a respite. When the medical provider
arrives, one of the issues she has to decide is what
medication to prescribe for Ms. F. While she is
there, Ms. F repeats her ritual so even the provider
has some understanding of the situation.

The medical provider knows that Ms. F is anxious, but she nevertheless has to decide whether to put her on medication to calm her
and change her behavior. The alternative is that the patient will be
cared for by short-tempered nurses or transferred to a nursing home
that is able to deal with "this kind of problem." Even if lucid,
patients such as Ms. F frequently are given no choice and in fact
might never know they are starting new medications.

Decision-making also can be removed from the elderly person
who "sundowns." As night approaches, these patients become confused and as a result wander aimlessly, start cooking, or simply
become frightened. The family requests sleeping medication for
them because they are worried about their safety, but cannot stay
up all night to monitor them. The sleeping medication is often
administered without the agreement or even knowledge of the
elderly patient.

A better solution would be a home health aid who could spend
several hours talking with elderly persons, walking with them, or
having a small snack. Providing such a resource would cost money,
but the side effects of sleeping medications also can lead to greater costs, financial and otherwise, as the following case demonstrates.

Mr. M, who is 84 years old and lives with his
son's family, does fine during the day but is active
at night. He explains that he does not require much
sleep and he just likes to "putter around." The

family once found him cooking at 1:00 a.m. and are worried that he will forget to turn off the stove if he does it again. Another time they discovered that he had taken a walk to a nearby park at 1:00 a.m.. Because they are concerned for his safety, they discuss the situation with Mr. M's medical provider, who prescribes a sleeping medication. One night, after having taken his sleeping pill, Mr. M becomes restless and decides to take a walk. Because the sleeping pill made him drowsy and unstable, he falls, fracturing his hip. He is in the hospital for three weeks, where he undergoes surgery to repair his hip and physical therapy.

Sleep patterns change with age—this is a normal part of growing old. Prescribing medication can simply magnify the problem, however. In addition to the morbidity and trauma they caused for Mr. M, sleeping pills can have rebound effects, for example, hallucinations. The immediate point, though, is that the failure to fund alternative ways of dealing with the problems of the elderly may be a false economy.

One of the most obvious responses to many problems of the elderly is better home care, yet society is unwilling to provide resources such as home health aids. Much could be accomplished by removing restrictions that currently inhibit the use of home care services and generally expanding the services that are available. A more drastic, but more desirable, solution would be to make home care the mandatory entry point into the health care system for elderly persons. In order for such a change to succeed, good assessments of patients and good rehabilitation services also would have to be provided. Where would the money be found? Either the health care budget would have to be increased, or funds would have to be diverted from the overwhelming proportion of the budget that goes to hospitals and high-technology care. Neither course appears politically palatable. But as long as prescribing medication remains the automatic response to problems of the elderly, because it is easy and because it appears cheap, better alternatives will not be pursued.

The Risks of Poly-Pharmacy

Elderly patients take an average of five different medications.[3] The dangers of multiple drugs are well recognized. Drugs can interact to reduce or negate the effect of one or more of them. On the other hand, the interaction can be synergistic, increasing the effect of a drug beyond that desired. In addition, recognizing side effects and identifying their causes becomes more difficult. An elderly patient might be taking a diuretic, a cardiac medication, an anti-inflammatory, and an antibiotic simultaneously. Each of these drugs can cause psychological changes such as depression and confusion, so the combination makes it exceedingly difficult to attribute a particular side effect to any one of them or to any combination of them.

The risk of toxic side effects also arises when prescription drugs are mixed with over-the-counter drugs. Patients with arthritis who are on anti-inflammatory drugs must be careful about taking aspirin, for example. Anti-inflammatory drugs are known to cause stomach upset, heartburn, headache, and dizziness in some people. A rarer, but more serious, side effect is bleeding from the stomach, and that can be exacerbated by aspirin. But a patient who has a headache or the flu might not suspect there is a danger of aspirin or a decongestant containing aspirin interacting with another drug because both are used so widely. The obvious remedy for this potential problem is public education combined with education by medical providers.

Side Effects

With geriatric patients there is a significant risk of iatrogenic problems from medications. Because these patients commonly have decreased renal function, side effects can occur at the recommended dosage of a drug for younger patients. As well, the existence of combination medications, a diuretic combined with an antihypertensive, for instance, makes it difficult to assess side effects. This problem is compounded by uncertainty as to whether a change is a side effect of a drug or a symptom of the patient's condition. For example, an 84-year-old woman's hypertension was not controlled by the diuretic she had been taking for a number of years, so her medical provider prescribed Aldomet. On her return visit three weeks later, her blood pressure was still not controlled, and, in addition, a lack of affect and mild depression were noted. Is the patient's depression a side effect of the Aldomet, or is it a consequence of the general deterioration of her health? Being uncertain of that, should her provider change her medication now, hoping that the patient's depression is caused by the drug, but knowing that she might create other problems for the patient by stopping and starting too many drugs in a short time, or should she simply monitor the patient more closely and give her more time to adjust to a new drug?

Confusion can be a major indicator of health problems in elderly patients, but it can also be caused by drugs. One danger is that iatrogenic confusion will be misinterpreted. A 78-year-old man broke his hip and was hospitalized. His family viewed his ensuing confusion as a sign of senility and inquired about the possibility of a nursing home placement. In fact, his confusion was the result of drugs and the hospital environment. Another danger is that confusion caused by a treatable disease will be attributed to a patient's medications.

Because the increased sensitivity of the elderly makes them susceptible to side effects, and because side effects are difficult to assess in the elderly, providers should be circumspect in their prescribing practices. Some providers feel that elderly patients should not take more than three or four prescription and non-prescription medications simultaneously because of the dangers of side effects.

Communication failures are evident in dealing with side effects. Geriatric patients can be reluctant to cause inconvenience to medi-

cal providers through repeated telephone calls about their problems, so they experiment instead. If a diuretic seems to be causing
frequent urination, the drug is taken less often or stopped. If a beta
blocker is perceived to be causing insomnia, it is stopped. Patients
convictions about the connection between behavior changes and
their medications can be quite rigid. If, at the next visit, the provider
explains that beta blockers do not cause insomnia, he or she might
not be believed. The provider then can prescribe a different beta
blocker or try to convince the patient to take the present beta blocker
by prescribing a sleeping pill to counteract the insomnia. But
changing medications or adding medications is not a panacea
because new drugs have to be monitored closely. That requires
more frequent visits, which the patient may be unwilling or unable
to make. In a nursing home closer monitoring demands more work
from the nurses, for example, taking urine specimens and blood
pressures and weighing patients more often. Such resistance forces
the provider to assess the significance of the side effect, and he or

Perhaps the most complex communication problems involve
the identification of side effects. A side effect might not be perceived to be a problem by a patient because of the patient's conception
of what a "normal" lifestyle for an elderly person is, as the following case demonstrates.

> Mr. R, who is 74 years old, has severe hyperten-
> sion and heart disease. With diuretic, antihyperten-
> sive, and cardiac medications his symptoms resolve
> and his blood pressure is lowered, but he realizes
> that he must continue these medications for the rest
> of his life. On repeated visits his medical provider
> notes that his blood pressure is not consistent and
> his edema and jugular venous distention vary, re-
> gardless of changes in his medications. His pro-
> vider suspects that Mr. R is noncompliant, but she
> cannot figure out why. Finally Mr. R reveals that he
> is impotent when he takes his medications accord-
> ing to directions. He has been embarrassed to men-

tion this problem because he assumes that a diag-
nois of cardiac disease means that one's sex life is
over.

Beta blockers can cause impotency, and sexual dysfunction can
be a particularly difficult issue with geriatric patients. Because they
assume that advancing age and an active sex life are incompatible,
they are inclined to accept side effects such as impotency rather
than raising them as problems. A man's partner may accept the
situation as well because she assumes that menopause means the
end of her sexual activity. In this situation, discovering what the
problem is and dealing with it is primarily an exercise in good communication. The age of the medical provider can be an obstacle
because a patient might feel uncomfortable discussing sensitive
issues with someone who is significantly younger. In any event the
provider must be knowledgeable about and sensitive to the changes
that occur as people grow older and must take an active role in
pursuing possible problems and deciphering what patients are
saying. A provider who passively accepts what patients say and
who deals only with problems that patients explicitly raise will
miss opportunities to improve their care.

Compliance

With a chronic regime of many different drugs, regardless of
whether they are taken once a day or four times a day, compliance
becomes a major problem for both the patient and the medical
provider. A home care patient might want to follow a medication
regimen closely, but be physically or mentally incapable of doing
so. Arthritic patients have difficulty opening the child-proof tops
that most pharmacies use as a safety precaution. A patient whose
vision is failing might be unable to read the label or might become
suspicious because the pills from the most recent prescription are
a different color, size, or shape. A patient who is forgetful can mistakenly think that he or she has not yet taken medications. A patient

who is mildly confused can mistakenly think that he or she has already taken medications. Both repeating doses and missing doses are common, and both occur despite the best intentions of the patient. The medical provider and pharmacist might have talked to the patient, but unless they know the patient and the home situation well and can anticipate these problems, non-compliance will remain a danger.

Poor communication between medical provider and patient is a recurrent cause of noncompliance. The introduction of cheaper generic drugs has made it more difficult to provide accurate and comprehensive yet intelligible information to patients. Patients can find it difficult to remember and pronounce the technical names of their medications, so they report that they are taking a blue pill for their arthritis and a water pill for their blood pressure, for example. They might recognize names such as "Motrin" and Diuril," but they can become confused when the names of their generic equivalents, "Ibuprofen" and "Chlorothiazide," start appearing on the labels of their prescriptions. Rather than asking questions, the patient, believing that the provider or pharmacist has made a mistake, might not take the drug. Or the patient might take both Motrin and Ibuprofen at home, assuming that a new drug has been prescribed. Such problems need to be anticipated and discussed with the patient so that the dangers of undertreatment and toxicity can be avoided.

Noncompliance that results from attempts to self-manage side effects is frequent in geriatric patients on long-term medications. A patient taking one diuretic a day might be bothered but not alarmed by the increased frequency of urination and the feeling of dry mouth the drug is causing. Taking the drug every second or third day instead of daily might make the side effects more tolerable, but it also might cause the drug to be ineffective in controlling hypertension. Again, this is a problem that needs to be foreseen and discussed with the patient.

Noncompliance can be risky for a home care patient because the "solution" can be nursing home placement. Patients in nursing homes lose their power to be noncompliant, if they wish, and to "soften" the side effects of drugs. A patient might refuse a drug that he or she feels is causing an undesirable side effect, but if the medical provider does not believe the side effect is associated with the drug, the patient's refusal probably will be overriden. A number of strategies exist to get nursing home patients to take medications. The medical provider and nurses can adjust the dose or change the drug. But more forceful techniques are available. Nurses dispense medications to patients, give them fluids to aid in swallowing, and even check their mouths to make sure drugs have been swallowed. Or nurses can try to disguise a drug by, for instance, crushing it in applesauce or dissolving it in fruit juice. Finally, if a drug is deemed essential, it can be given by injection.

Yet placement in a nursing home sometimes is necessary. Hypertensive patients who forget to take their medications, for example, can have very high or fluctuating blood pressure that results in a transient ischemic attack (TIA) or a minor heart attack. If a TIA occurs, the patient could suffer a minor cut or bruise, but more serious injury such as a fractured hip could ensue. If the prospective harm is sufficiently great, and if no less drastic alternatives are available, a placement may be justified, even over the patient's objection. But moving a patient to a nursing home can easily become an indiscriminate "solution" to genuine problems of noncompliance, as well as a spurious solution to other problems for which noncompliance serves as a symptom or an excuse.

Patients who do not live in institutions obviously have greater control over the medications they take, and their noncompliance, even if foolish or irrational, is not overriden. Noncompliance on the part of these patients often results from an inability to understand the nature of chronic disease or an unwillingness to accept it. An 84-year-old man, although without symptoms, was diagnosed as having heart disease, and medication that would help prevent the onset of symptoms was prescribed. The man did not understand the medical jargon used by his provider, however, so he was not convinced of the need for medication. Instead of asking questions or saying he would not take the medicine, he left the office and never filled the prescription. Similarly, a 68-year-old woman who was supposed to take three pills a day for hypertension stopped them because she believed that she could feel when her blood pressure was high and that drinking a cup of herb tea at that time lowered it. If her blood pressure did not feel elevated, she had no reason to take pills daily; moreover, she was spared the expense and the side effects of the drug.

Chronic disease can be difficult to accept because of the changes in lifestyle it entails. Adult onset diabetes can require changes in a diet that may have been established for 60 years. Stress incontinence can prevent a patient from going on outings longer than an hour, such as shopping or to a movie, for fear that a cough might cause a loss of control of urine. Patients with newly diagnosed chronic diseases such as hypertension and diabetes that are not yet controlled can cancel or shorten vacations for fear of being away from their medical providers. The real fear, however, is loss of control over one's life. For example, a 76-year-old woman with adult onset diabetes did everything her medical provider advised— she went on a strict diet and increased her daily walking and lost ten pounds—but her urine and blood sugar tests indicated that she would still need an oral hypoglycemic. To many patients it does not seem "fair" to have to take medications for the rest of their lives. Again, allowing patients to participate in decisions concerning the management of their chronic diseases seems to be the best response. Participation requires education, and better understanding of diseases could lead to better compliance. Participation also restores control, and more control could lead to better compliance.

Compliance always will be a problem, as anyone who has tried to take antibiotics four times a day for 10 days will appreciate. Elderly patients are often on chronic regimens of multiple medications, some of which are taken once, some twice, and some three or four times a day, so the problem is formidable. Mechanical devices help. An arthritic patient could use a pushbutton releaser for containers; a forgetful patient could be given daily divided doses;

and a visually impaired patient could have divided daily doses set up for a week. But communication and responsibility remain essential. A health care educator could help patients understand their chronic diseases and why lifelong medication regimens are necessary. The hope is that instilling responsibility and control in the patient will breed compliance.

Financial Constraints

The overwhelming cost of medicine to elderly persons living on modest pensions and savings sometimes forces them to make choices about their health. An 82-year-old woman with diabetes mellitus and increased blood pressure, for example, visited her medical provider only every six months to a year. Even when her provider explained to her that her diabetes was poorly controlled and with the new medication being prescribed closer monitoring would be necessary, she failed to make the two-week return visit. When she finally did come back to the clinic, she explained that she had difficulty paying for her prescriptions so she had to decide either to visit her provider at six-month intervals rather than the recommended two-week intervals or to buy her medicines. Both alternatives are risky. The new medication might not work, but monitoring is necessary to determine whether it is effective. On the other hand, monitoring is pointless if the patient is not taking the medication. The patient has chosen the reasonable course dictated by her limited finances, but she should not have to make this decision.

The lack of a private medical provider, because of financial difficulties, can create prescribing problems through the practice of hospital or provider "hopping." A patient who depends upon outpatient departments or emergency wards for medical care is subject to multiple prescribers who, in virtue of the acute, episodic care they provide, are unlikely to be aware of the other providers a patient has seen and the complete set of medications the patient is taking. Following the advice of multiple prescribers creates the danger of toxic drug interactions, as the following case illustrates.

>   Ms. N, who is 78 years old, comes to her provider to have her high blood pressure and diabetes monitored. The provider instructs her to return with all the medications she is taking. When Ms. N comes back in a week, she has a bag with 25 bottles of medication. The labels indicate that some are old, some are duplicates, and some are different drugs used to treat the same problem. Ms. N has been taking these medications haphazardly. She has visited the emergency department of a local hospital on several occasions, possibly for problems created by the combination of drugs she took that week.

The ideal situation is for patients to have continous, comprehensive primary care delivered by one medical provider, but financial limitations make that ideal impossible for a significant number of elderly persons. Although Medicare pays for hospital and office visists and for diagnostic testing, there is an annual deductible. This out-of-pocket expense can be such a strain on the incomes of elderly persons that they avoid routine visits to their providers for as long as possible every new fiscal year. As a result their overall quality of care suffers, and individual problems are treated only when they become more serious than they should. With such patients their first visit for care every fiscal year is to an emergency room, which can involve an ambulance ride, consultations in the emergency department, and X-rays and laboratory tests. Payment of the deductible is postponed but not avoided, and the result is medical care that is more expensive for the health care system and more traumatic for the patient. The patient could be admitted to the hospital, but in any event is likely to leave with a number of prescriptions either duplicating or adding to those drugs already at home. The attempt to save money through the annual Medicare deductible can in fact create greater costs to the system both in the short term and in the long term if the patient's health deteriorates as a result of the delay in seeking care.

Problems for Dying Patients

The Locus of Decision-Making

An elderly person's right to participate in decisions concerning medications can become the right to decide to die when medications are necessary to preserve life. The issue of refusing life-saving treatment has been extensively discussed, but usually in the context of acute, high-technology, tertiary care. Two cases that involve the refusal of commonplace medications in a chronic care environment will be used simply to reinforce points.

> Ms. W, a 94-year-old nursing home patient, is alert and oriented. She is noted, however, to have decreased appetite and increased lethargy. A clinical examination reveals that she has pneumonia. Her medical provider assures her that with antibiotics she will get better. Ms. W nevertheless requests that all medication be withheld. She explains that she has had a good, long life and her time now has come. She asks her provider to please let her die. But the majority of Ms. W's medical team feels that she is depressed because she is sick. They argue that antibiotic treatment is not invasive and that health care personnel have a duty to use such minimal means to preserve life. Ms. W is given the antibiotics, and her condition improves. When her provider visits Ms. W after she has recovered, she asks Ms.

> W if she is happy that her wish was denied. Ms. W
> reaffirms her request that treatment be withheld if
> she again contracts pneumonia.

In Ms. W's case the decision of a competent patient was over-
ridden because it was believed to be an irrational product of the
depression caused by her illness and because it conflicted with the
health care providers' perceived professional duty. The former
reason was not borne out by Ms. W's reassertion that treatment be
withheld in the future. The latter reason rests on the dubious pro-
position that the professional duty to use routine, simple, non-invasive treatments outweighs the patient's clearly expressed desire.

In the next case health care professionals are forced to make a
decision on behalf of an incompetent patient.

> Ms. P, who is 84 years old, has been severely se-
> nile, incontinent, and arthritic for more than six
> years. Decreased appetite and fever are noted, and
> a clinical examination reveals pneumonia. Because
> Ms. P has no family, the medical team discusses her
> case and decides to withhold treatment because her
> quality of life is so poor. They see no reason to
> prolong her life when pneumonia can be a painless
> way to die. Ms. P slips into a coma and dies four
> days later.

Presumably Ms. P's medical team does not accept the professional duty to use simple, noninvasive means to treat pneumonia in all
cases. Ms. P's past and future quality of life seem more important
to them.

The status of a medical intervention as routine, ordinary, and
noninvasive still plays an important role in the decision making of
health care professionals. As Ms. W's plight reveals, it can be
regarded as more important than the right of a competent patient to
decide whether to accept treatment. With the exception of chemo-

therapy and experimental drugs, administering medications is not regarded by health care professionals as a distinct "procedure," such as an operation, to which a patient must expressly consent. Instead it is viewed as an obligatory part of routine medical care, and the wishes of the patient are not accorded the same seriousness they would have if an operation, however minor, were in question.

The status of a medical intervention as routine, ordinary, or non-invasive does not carry the moral weight that health care professionals are disposed to attribute to it. As the two cases illustrate, the result of not administering an antibiotic can be as serious as the result of not performing a heart transplant. Instead, the consequences for the patient carry most of the moral weight and give so much moral significance to the patient's wishes. This is not a novel point, but it bears repeating in the context of prescribing commonplace medications, regardless of whether they are life-saving.

Pain Control

Assuring dying patients that they will have effective pain control also has been much discussed. At the level of the individual patient, the element of clinical judgment in prescribing pain control medications is inescapable. Evaluating pain in a comatose patient is often difficult. Is moaning a reliable sign of pain? Is the absence of a "peaceful" look on the patient's face sufficient to diagnose pain? Patients with cancer are routinely assumed to require pain medication, but what about patients with pneumonia, dehydration, congestive heart failure, or cerebralvascular accidents?

Pain medications can cause hallucinations, vomiting, disorientation, and decreased respiration and heart rate, any of which could accelerate death. The failure to provide sufficient pain medication, whatever the dosage required, is difficult to justify, however, even when the consequence may be expedited death. Fear of malpractice litigation, personal anxieties about death, the worry that the patient might become addicted, and the increased work that counting narcotics on every shift entails for nurses are all otiose reasons. To some extent, the issue is empirical. Is heroin really more effective than morphine in controlling pain? Would the legalization of heroin for pain control really make the drug more easily available in communities at a time when society is waging war on recreational drug use? But on balance it is difficult to see how prudential, emotional, and political considerations and empirical uncertainty, even collectively, can be more important than providing effective palliative care to dying patients. What, ultimately, is the price of mercy?

Conclusion

Hagar Shipley, the 90-year-old protagonist in Margaret Laurence's novel, *The Stone Angel*, muses to herself:

> The door of my room has no lock. They say it is because I might get taken ill in the night, and then how could they get in to tend me (*tend*—as though I were a crop, a cash crop). So they may enter my room any time they choose. Privacy is a privilege not granted to the aged or the young. Sometimes very young children can look at the old, and a look passes between them, conspiratorial, sly and knowing. It's because neither are human to the middling ones, those in their prime, as they say, like beef.[4]

This reflection captures, better than any philosophical essay could, the main moral problem in providing health care to the elderly. Individuals who have been responsible for themselves and their families for most of their lives are disfranchised by age, regardless of whether doing so is warranted by infirmity. They move from being responsible to being an obligation. Because the obligation to take care of them devolves on others, their lives are controlled by others and open to others. Because taking care of them is an obligation, it can be regarded as a burden that is undertaken grudgingly. The attitude that taking care of the elderly is society's obligation helps to explain why decision-making responsibility is removed from the elderly and why funding for their needs is not more generous.

This change in the status of the elderly is particularly pernicious because it is subtle. Families and health care professionals can be unaware that such a shift in attitude has occurred. They simply assume that a person who is old needs to be protected and taken care of by others. The problems that arise with respect to prescribing medications flow, in large measure, from this general attitude toward the elderly. Their solution depends, in large measure, upon adopting a more enlightened attitude.

References

[1]G. H. Kramer (1985) Cost effectiveness implications based on a comparison of nursing home and home care mix. *Health Serv. Res.* **20**, 387–405.

[2]S. Bachrach (1982) Who lives in nursing homes? Unpublished manuscript.

[3]R. J. Master et al. (1980) A continuum of care for the inner city. *New Engl. J. Med. 302*, 1434–1440.

[4]M. Laurence (1964) *The Stone Ange,l* McClelland and Stewart, Toronto, p.4.

Prescribing Drugs
for the Aged and Dying

Ron Yezzi

Introduction

In the treatment of the aged and dying, decisions about drugs tend to be overshadowed by questions about the general goals of care for terminal patients and by more dramatic issues such as the use of resuscitation, feeding tubes, and respirators. Yet prescribing drugs is almost always an essential part of total patient care and is thus worthy of special comment. Drugs are often vital to preserving life and controlling pain. Perhaps they may even provide a proper means of ending life. This latter possibility becomes a matter of serious ethical debate as more patients resort to drastic measures to ensure an ending to their lives—such as storing and hiding pills for later use, pulling out respirator tubes, and using firearms.

The elderly frequently use prescription drugs. Although constituting about 10 percent of the population in the United States, the elderly account for about 23 percent of total drug consumption. They tend to be more subject to adverse drug reactions than the population generally. And since they may well be taking more than one prescription drug, the consequent drug interactions exacerbate the reaction problem. The elderly also face special problems using drugs properly. Failing eyesight, faulty memory, and a greater propensity to seek home remedies or popularly advertised "cures" may lessen their compliance with a prescription. As a result, problems

31

arise for conscientious, concerned physicians. We can also reasonably infer that dying patients present many similar problems. Since the problems mentioned, however, require primarily practical solutions rather than ethical policy decisions, we will not consider them here.

In discussing drugs specifically, we also want to retain a proper perspective on total care. Health care entails much more than biochemistry. So the issue of prescribing drugs cannot be seen independently of the general goals of care. Patients need our humane concern and deserve as much comfort as possible. Accordingly, they have emotional, social, physical, and environmental needs that should be addressed along with any use of prescription drugs.

For our purposes here, we will not deal with all the elderly. We will use the term "the aged" in a special way, not to be confused with general discussions of the "wisdom of the aged" or with general discussions of worthwhile contributions that the elderly still can make. We want to focus upon the elderly in a state of *dependence*. Accordingly, we will take *the aged* to include those elderly patients who, by reason of irreversible mental and/or physical impairment, require constant or near-constant care. Similarly, we will take *the dying* to include those patients who, by reason of an irreversible life-ending disease, are beyond cure through techniques of contemporary medicine. We will also assume that we are dealing with patients in a sufficiently immediate state of decline as to cause especially agonizing questions for health care deciders.

To limit the scope of the inquiry, we will avoid questions regarding use of placebos and experimental drugs—although these are admittedly significant issues. We will also take the step of not worrying about what the laws presently require. So, if laws in the United States ban "mercy killing" or heroin use in general medical practice, this will not affect our considerations. We will simply proceed on the assumption that laws should institutionalize whatever analysis establishes as a morally best position.

I plan to treat the issues involved in five stages—considering (1) conditions that apply to the aged and dying, (2) the types of drugs available for treatment, (3) a brief survey of relevant ethical principles, (4) ethical decisions in prescribing drugs, and (5) guidelines in prescribing drugs for the aged and dying.

Patient Conditions

The aged and dying (along with everyone else) have particular fears about an irreversible, debilitating state of dependence based upon a perceived deterioration in the quality of their lives. Aside from economically based conditions, the major fears include loss of the ability to move about, incontinence, mental disability, pain, abandonment, and loss of normal functions such as the ability to communicate, to feed oneself, to provide personal hygiene (bathing, shaving, hair grooming, and so on). For most patients, these fears become especially acute because they see themselves as having lost what they once had and treasured.

We want to consider these patients with respect to use of drugs when these fears are realized. Their mental and/or physical impairments may be moderate or severe. Their condition may be deteriorating slowly or more rapidly; other serious medical problems may or may not arise; there can be varying degrees of pain. Treatment alternatives will vary according to what conditions apply to a given patient. But by considering several test cases, it is hoped we can get a better grasp of some major ethical problems that arise.

Case 1

On January 5, 1986, CBS' *60 Minutes* broadcast a story covering the apparently growing acceptance of euthanasia in Holland. One patient, a 63-year-old woman, is almost totally paralyzed with multiple sclerosis—from which she has suffered for a number of years. So far, her husband has taken care her, and she has been content with that. But he has a serious heart condition and may not live much longer. There was no mention of any other family members able or willing to take care of her. She has always opposed going to a nursing home. Several years ago, she signed a living will instructing her physician to end her life by administering a lethal injection if her husband should die. Her present prognosis indicates that she can live several more years, with appropriate care. Her physician points out that she was quite depressed before, but that she has been much happier since signing the living will—knowing that she has a way of ending her suffering at what she considers to be the appropriate time. Is administering a lethal injection according to this patient's wishes ethically acceptable? Note that she is mentally competent, has maintained the same wishes for several years, and is suffering from a severely debilitating, terminal disease.

Case 2

The next is a case of Alzheimer's disease. The patient, a former telephone company executive forced to retire at age 58 because of early signs of the disease, has reached a point where spouse, family and friends are no longer recognized, speech has deteriorated so that miscellaneous monosyllables are the only sounds, incontinence is present, and the patient is no longer able to walk. The patient also is being treated for hypertension. The prognosis is coma and death. After a long seven-year struggle with the disease, the spouse wishes only that the tragedy would end. According to the spouse and family, the patient frequently made clear earlier in life fears of dying a debilitating death and being a burden on everyone—although in fighting off and denying the early symptoms of Alzheimer's disease, the patient never took steps to sign a living will or inform the doctor of any personal wishes regarding long-term treatment. The patient currently has pneumonia, and the spouse requests that no antibiotics be used. The spouse also wonders whether it might be better to discontinue the treatment for hypertension—with a consequent increase in the likelihood of stroke or heart failure—if the patient survives the pneumonia. What should the doctors prescribe? In contrast with Case 1, note that this patient is mentally *in*competent, with the prior wishes about treatment not entirely clearcut.

Case 3

This patient, 73 years old, is in the final stages of cancer, with the likelihood of considerable pain. The prognosis indicates that the patient has perhaps six months to live, at most. The patient refuses radiation treatment and chemotherapy, demanding instead to be treated with laetrile, a drug considered worthless by the medical profession. For controlling pain, the patient wants to be sure that doctors will provide maximum pain relief, even if the dosages hasten death. In addition, the patient asks whether heroin might be used as the pain-killer — having heard that heroin is routinely and effectively used at hospices in Britain. The patient is lucid and mentally competent, although already experiencing some pain. The family strongly supports these requests. This case differs from the previous two primarily in the way the patient wants to actively direct drug treatment. Should physicians acquiesce to the patient's requests?

Case 4

This 75-year-old patient suffers from organic brain syndrome. In addition to occasional lapses into confusion, the patient exhibits paranoia. As a result, those concerned with long-term care find the patient difficult to deal with. Some psychotropic drug seems to be in order. But different drugs will have different effects on the patient. In particular, some have a more sedating effect than others. The patient's condition is deteriorating and the patient shows no interest in any constructive activities. Heavy sedation would make it much easier for the staff to provide care. What should be prescribed? This case differs from the others in that the doctors must decide to what extent they are going to reduce the patient's capacity for autonomy.

Drug Treatments Available

Drugs prescribed for the aged and the dying can serve a variety of purposes, as the outline below shows:

I. Life-preserving drugs
   A. Therapeutic
      1. For curative purposes (e.g., antibiotics to treat infection or chemotherapy to cure cancer)
      2. For maintenance purposes (e.g., thiazides to treat hypertension or chemotherapy to prolong life)
   B. Experimental
II. Mood-altering drugs
   A. For pain control
   B. For psychiatric syndromes
      1. Depression
      2. Paranoia
      3. Organic brain syndrome
III. Life-ending drugs

Under therapeutic drugs, we usually mean those of proven treatment effectiveness. We should point out, however, that there are two special, more questionable classes of drugs regarded by some to be therapeutic—namely, those generally regarded by the medical profession to be worthless (e.g., laetrile) and those regarded to be unproven for use in a particular country (e.g., a drug used in Europe, but not approved for use in the US by the FDA).

Serving these various purposes raises some important ethical issues.

For example, a drug used in sufficient dosage to control pain may also hasten death and, hence, in some sense, becomes a life-ending drug. Suppose, however, that the physician denies any intention to hasten death—arguing that the purpose for the drug dosage is the control of pain, thereby bringing comfort to a terminal patient. Does a statement of intention of this sort establish that any hastening of death is an unintended secondary effect? And even if it does, how can we establish that this is the physician's *real* intention, rather than any desire to hasten death?

The hospice movement, in particular, has taken the lead in stressing the need for effective pain control in caring for terminal patients. And in Britain, the home of the hospice movement, there has been considerable stress on the use of morphine and heroin (diamorphine) in pain-control. Some British physicians, commenting on medicine in the US, suggest that too timid use of morphine and a refusal to use heroin cause unnecessary pain to terminal patients. To what extent should narcotics be used in pain control?

If use of life-ending drugs is morally acceptable, should the patient take pills or receive a lethal injection? Taking pills allows the patient rather than the doctor to be the one bringing about death. This would seem more in keeping with preserving the patient's autonomy, while also relieving medical personnel of emotional and instrumental burdens. On the other hand, lethal injection under close medical supervision seems to be a more reliable method. In the program on *60 Minutes*, one Dutch doctor said that pills were only 80 percent effective. He preferred performing this treatment under surgical conditions, using barbiturates followed by use of curare.

Ethical Considerations

Various ethical considerations can affect our judgments regarding the prescribing of various kinds of drugs for the aged and dying. There follows a brief summary of several principles that are reasonable enough to command widespread support among health care providers and ethicists. Disagreements, when they arise, are much more likely to occur as disputes over the priority and application of the principles rather than in their acceptance or rejection. Although a more elaborate set of principles would contribute to a fuller account, the five principles listed here should be sufficient to provide some conclusions for the test cases already mentioned.

1. *Autonomy: As much as is reasonably possible, health care providers should respect patient autonomy.*

Autonomy, or self-governance, is a fundamental value because it enhances our dignity as human beings and increases the quality of our lives. In addition, we see the freedom to make our own choices about our life to be a fundamental right. In health care, the principle entails that patients have a great deal to say about the course of their treatment.

Of course, we have to recognize that not all decisions are autonomous, and paternalistic action is sometimes acceptable. Accordingly, we need some standards that establish whether or not a decision is autonomous. Moreover, we want standards that hold up in the context of serious health care decisions. That is to say, we want standards stricter than those by which we casually regard most ordinary decisions in everyday life to be autonomous. From the literature on the subject, we can glean the following primary standard: A patient's decision is *autonomous* if a representative rational person would regard the decision (a) to be the result of reasonable, informed deliberation and (b) to be reasonably judged to be in the patient's best interest. (Note that the requirement of *reasonableness* does not demand that one choose the best, most rational alternative. The decision must be reasonable enough to be defensible to rational persons.) To this primary standard, we can add the secondary one that decisions that fit coherently into the patient's past history or are held over longer periods of time are more convincing expressions of autonomy.

According to these standards, we should grant that even a decision to end one's life can, *at least sometimes*, be autonomous. I have known numerous rational persons who, having studied and deliberated upon the issue of terminal illness, have concluded that a speedy death would sometimes be in a patient's best interest—

whether the patient be themselves or others. And I do not think my report is at all unusual. To be sure, we cannot take so irreversible a step lightly. But we have to include it as a possibility within the range of autonomous actions.

2. *Avoidance of Harm: Health care providers should not inflict harm on a patient without compensating benefit.*

Although we ordinarily want to characterize any health care procedure in positive terms, as a benefit for the patient, we take the dictum, "do no harm," as being even more basic. "Harm," *interpreted as injury or pain*, seems to be more concrete, more easily identifiable than "benefit" in medical practice—especially in the case of the aged and dying where the hoped for benefits seem very limited, relatively insignificant, and less probable than the prospects of real injury and pain. Thus physicians, if they must err, are exhorted to err on the side of caution. It is better to avoid harm than to take excessive risks to achieve hoped for benefits.

3. *Sanctity of Life: Health care providers should respect the sanctity of human life.*

Respect for the sanctity of life requires that we go to great lengths to preserve life. This respect is a basic value in a health care provider's commitment to medicine. Thus it is not surprising that they are reluctant to let their patients go. Nor is it surprising that this reluctance usually turns into repulsion at the thought of administering a lethal injection to a patient. No matter how sensible or reasonable such an act may seem in some situations, it still "goes against the grain."

Nevertheless, the sanctity of life principle does not seem to entail an absolute obligation to preserve life at all costs—since the complete elimination of quality of life considerations, which an absolute obligation would entail, does not have much support even among those strongly committed to the sanctity of life principle.

4. *Acceptance of Death: At some point, patients, family, and*
        health care providers should show acceptance of the
        reality of disease and death.

As much as we revere the sanctity of life, we also must accept the
reality of disease and death. And at some point in the progress of
disease, we must direct our efforts toward preparing for death rather
than simply trying to preserve life. This principle sets a goal for
both the patient and others involved in the decision-making. What
treatment is appropriate, of course, requires other ethical considerations. Nevertheless, we cannot let a refusal to accept death
interfere with our consideration of treatment alternatives.

5. *Others' Interests: The legitimate interests of others beside*
        the patient should be considered in any decision-making
        process.

Although the patient's interests are rightly the focus of concern,
one cannot go very far in the decision-making process without
taking account of the legitimate interests of others. Thus, we need
to avoid a tendency to denigrate others' interests as a crass interference with the rights of patients. Physicians have the right to act
according to their knowledge and conscience; family members
have a right to consideration of their wishes, suffering, and the
strain on their resources; and society has a right to protect its larger
interests regarding the allocation of resources and the impact of a
particular patient's case on others.

It is interesting to note how often both sides on an issue will appeal to others' interests to support their position. If those who fav-
or preserving life cannot make much of a case in terms of benefits
to the patient or respect for life, they usually argue that hastening
death, even when it is most reasonable for the patient, sets a bad
precedent for society and paves the way for abuses. And if those
who favor hastening death cannot make much of a case in terms of
the patient's decision and avoiding harm, they usually appeal to
interests of the family or society.

Principles 1 and 2 assert the patient's interests solely and directly; principles 3 and 4 assert the interests of both the patient and others; and principle 5 asserts the interests of others solely and directly. If we assign the principles roughly equal weight in decision-making, we achieve a reasonable balance with the patient's interest still being the primary focus of concern.

At this point, we are ready to consider the test cases previously mentioned in order to formulate some guidelines for prescribing drugs for the aged and the dying. For the first test case, we will consider each ethical principle separately to better understand its application. For the other cases, we will provide a briefer account—relying on the applications for the first test case and adding appropriate analysis as needed.

Case 1: The Patient with Multiple Sclerosis

Autonomy

We want to know: Can this patient—in requesting a lethal injection should her husband die—satisfy the primary and secondary standards that establish that a decision is autonomous? More information about her decision would be helpful. From what we are given, however—that she is mentally competent and has held to the same decision for several years—we should be strongly inclined to judge her to be functioning autonomously. Having suffered from the disease for a number of years, she presumably is quite familiar with its pathology. In her decision, she rejects the alternative of going to a nursing home. This rejection may raise some question about how informed her deliberation is—considering that numerous elderly persons may be fearful about entering nursing homes only to find out after admission that their fears were caused by misapprehensions. On the other hand, we can also see how it is quite reasonable to reject the nursing home alternative on the grounds that it takes her out of the family environment where she feels comfortable and places her in a different one with the prospect of a lower quality of life as her condition worsens. It is hard to see how the nursing home provides benefits to her that so outweigh costs that we can deny the autonomy of her decision. Also, we should note that the nursing home alternative seems to have depressed her, whereas the alternative of the lethal injection apparently has not.

In this case, the woman should not have to prove that she will be unhappy in the nursing home or that the costs will outweigh the benefits. Rather the burden of proof lies with those who want to contravene her decision. If they want to say that her judgment about her prospective life in a nursing home is not properly informed and that there are considerable benefits that she does not foresee, then they have to show this. Moreover, if the woman is placed in the nursing home, they must continue to show that these benefits exist and that the woman recognizes them. Otherwise, they are not showing proper respect for her autonomy.

We can also point out that, generally, a patient deciding autonomously is given the right to refuse treatment. But if the sorts of reasons that the patient uses to refuse treatment are no better than, or different from, those that the patient uses to request treatment that will terminate life, there is, on the face of it, no reason to regard the latter decision as less autonomous than the former one.

Avoidance of Harm

Given this patient's condition and wish, it is difficult to see how one can force her to go on living without violating the "avoidance of harm" principle. Presumably, the woman is the best judge of the extent of her misery. There is a strong case for asserting that she can satisfy the standards of autonomy; and interference with her autonomy can reasonably be labeled a type of harm in itself. Moreover, the present state and prognosis of her disease make it difficult to find some compensating benefit in prolonging her life. What degree of assurance is there that the nursing home has the resources to improve her quality of life significantly?

Perhaps one can argue that death constitutes irreversible, ultimate harm and thus that the avoidance of harm principle requires prolonging life as long as possible. But relatively few people will agree. The frequency with which reasonable persons conclude that some extremely ill patients are fortunate to die quickly rather than slowly undermines the death-as-ultimate-harm argument.

Sanctity of Life

Respect for the sanctity of human life would seem to work against any ending of her life through lethal injection. We should not take this commitment to human life lightly. But we also need to be careful not to work with too simple an interpretation. Since the sanctity-of-life principle does not entail an absolute obligation to preserve life at all costs, quality of life considerations may establish that the principle in this case is best served by not prolonging life.

We would still, however, have to deal with that repulsion likely to arise at the prospect of a lethal injection. Given respect for the sanctity-of-life, it would take serious ethical considerations to overcome the repulsion.

Acceptance of Death

In this case, the patient is ready to accept death, and her judgment seems reasonable enough. The problem seems to be that of ensuring that others in the decision-making process do not let a refusal to accept death interfere with their doing what is best for the patient.

Others' Interests

The most troubling doubts regarding her request for a lethal injection arise in the consideration of other persons' interests.

The doctor, being the one who would administer the lethal injection, has a legitimate interest in the decision-making process. Even if physicians are convinced that the lethal injection is morally correct, many of them would still find their "treatment" difficult to accept, as already noted. Medical practitioners are committed to using their skills to preserve life, not to end it. Moreover, although a lethal injection will terminate the patient's consideration of the decision, doctors will have to live with their decisions for a much longer period—for the rest of their lives. The problem posed by lethal injections is probably evident when we consider that most of us would not require physicians to administer lethal injections against their conscience—no matter how much we may be convinced of the moral acceptability of the injection in some instances.

For reasons of this sort, it may seem more reasonable to have the patient take the most active part in ending life. The physician could prescribe pills, e.g., cyanide tablets, that patients would take themselves. Such a procedure would be more in keeping with allowing the patient to act autonomously; patients would be dying their own death rather than dying at the physician's hands. The procedure would also be closer to a situation in which physicians are simply forgoing the use of life-preserving treatment, a situation generally considered to be more acceptable. Taking this approach would accommodate the interests of physicians better than lethal injections.

This same line of reasoning might also seem to justify the physician staying out of the situation altogether. Physicians could simply leave it to their patients to find their own means of ending their lives. But this alternative presents two sorts of problems: (a) some patients may be incapable of finding suitable means and (b) some patients will "botch the job" with a consequent increase in misery for themselves. These problems raise serious questions about whether the patient is getting adequate care. Another alternative might be to have trained paramedical personnel, not physicians, administer the lethal injection. Although this might ease the burdens on physicians, it would in no way affect our deliberations here— since we are concerned with prescribing drugs for the aged and dying regardless of who happens to be administering them.

Society's interests are also important. Allowing a lethal injection here sets a precedent for other situations. In particular, it is hard to see how the procedure would not be extended to patients who do not voluntarily choose it. The extension is likely because the same sort of hopelessness evident in this woman's life is also present, perhaps even more so, in some other patients. Consider, for example, the case of a 93-year-old, bedridden patient in an advanced state of senile dementia, who has not recognized family members for several years, does not communicate with anyone in a significant way, and shows no interest in anything. Stress on the importance of autonomy in the decision-making process may seem to prevent the extension. Someone can argue that a life-ending drug should only be used if a terminal patient, acting autonomously, chose it. The problem, however, is that the primary standard for determining autonomy is not one of spontaneous free choice. Rather it requires reasonably informed deliberation and reasonable judgments of best interests—requirements of reasonableness that involve assessment of conditions very much like those existing in some nonautonomous patients. That is to say, what allows us to pronounce the patient's decision reasonable and therefore autonomous is recognition of a terminal debilitating disease that confines the patient to an extremely low quality of life; and this same condition can be present in nonautonomous patients. One can *almost* presume consent on the part of the nonautonomous patient—which may then justify use of the life-ending drug.

Consideration of others' interests raises some strong doubts about lethal injections; however, it does not point solely in the direction of rejecting their use. As soon as we consider allocation of resources, we can question the wisdom or justice in a decision to keep a hopelessly ill patient alive against the person's wishes in a situation that severely taxes the emotional, financial, and service resources of others.

Conclusion

In this case, we should allow use of a prescription drug to end this woman's life—although allowing her to do so by taking pills is preferable to the lethal injection. The principles of automomy, avoidance of harm, and acceptance of death justify this solution. The doubts raised in terms of sanctity of life and others' interests are not sufficient to negate this conclusion—especially since we can take measures that take into account our concerns for others' interests. For example, using pills (or some other self-administered technique) allows the patient, rather than the physician, to bring about death. A conscience clause would allow a physician to transfer the patient to another doctor rather than have to inject the lethal drug, or even prescribe the pills, oneself. Restrictions would prevent or at least limit extension of these procedures to certain classes of patients. Use of life-ending drugs might be simply banned in cases in which patient autonomy is lacking and no determination of intentions about treatment are determinable.

Would this conclusion also justify having carried out a request for lethal injection by the patient several years earlier? Given the conditions stated here, we should be inclined to answer negatively—since her husband was available to provide care and her situation was better in terms of quality of life. Would this conclusion also justify carrying out an autonomous request for a lethal injection by a much younger patient who happens to be in an almost identical situation as this woman patient? Each case has to be decided on its own merits. But we cannot rule out this particular possibility.

We may not accept the conclusion with enthusiasm; but we should find it better than the alternatives. Of course, we want full background information in a particular case; and we want to be sure that all reasonable alternatives are considered. Nevertheless, we still arrive at the conclusion that the five ethical principles considered justify carrying out some autonomous persons' requests for use of a drug that brings about death. Moreover, to deny these requests when it means that patients will resort to other measures, less likely to be effective or often more violent (such as overdosing on tranquilizers or putting a gun to the head), raises serious questions about whether or not the medical profession is providing proper care.

Other Cases

Case 2: *The Alzheimer's Disease Patient*

We should be able to settle one issue here quickly and simply. Should the treatment with a prescription drug for hypertension be discontinued? To withdraw a prescription for the purpose of causing some new medical complication for the patient violates the avoidance of harm principle flagrantly. Any goal to be achieved by such withdrawal can be achieved more effectively and acceptably by some other means. So no compensating benefit or other ethical principle would justify the withdrawal.

Now what can we say about the withholding of antibiotics to treat the pneumonia? In important ways, this patient is worse off than the one with multiple sclerosis—with mental capacity and ability to communicate having deteriorated grievously. Moreover, withholding antibiotics creates fewer ethical dilemmas and complications than the prescribing of a lethal drug. Accordingly, many of the same reasons that justified the conclusion there apply equally well and perhaps with stronger effect here—with the important exception, of course, of the autonomy issue. That is what we need to address.

Autonomy

In assessing autonomy in hastening of death situations, we can distinguish at least five classes of patients:

1. Presently autonomous patients who choose to hasten death.
2. Patients who cannot act autonomously now, but who acted autonomously in the past in signing a living will directing the hastening of death.
3. Patients who cannot act autonomously now and did not sign a living will previously, but who made clear informally or through lifestyle a wish to hasten death in situations of hopeless, terminal disease.

4. Patients whose wishes regarding the hastening of death in situations of hopeless, terminal disease are indeterminable.
5. Patients in any of the conditions described in 1, 2, and 3 who reject the hastening of death.

The Alzheimer's patient fits into class 3 or 4. The spouse and family place the patient in class 3, and they are likely to know more about the patient's prior attitudes and fears than anyone else. On the other hand, they may be reporting on attitudes and fears expressed in the distant past that are no longer relevant now; or they may be projecting *their own* frustration and despair into their reports regarding the patient. Even if we can alleviate these doubts about assigning the patient to class 3, we still must recognize that, in terms of a clear certification of an autonomous action, class 3 falls far short of 1 and 2. Thus the autonomy principle is not as relevant to a decision here as it was in the case of the multiple sclerosis patient.

Conclusion

Unless the physicians can definitely determine that the patient would not want treatment, they should use antibiotics because time is pressing and the patient's wishes are unclear. Not being able to appeal to an autonomous decision to forgo treatment in this case has serious implications in applying our five ethical principles. The inapplicability of the principle of autonomy is clear. But, in addition, we *cannot* say that the treatment with antibiotics violates the avoidance-of-harm principle simply by contravening the patient's wishes (as was assertable in the multiple sclerosis case). And, in terms of others' interests, there are the risks for society involved in setting precedents for hastening death without patient consent.

This conclusion concerning what physicians should do now, however, does not settle questions of long-term care. If at any time it should be possible to determine more clearly what the patient's wishes, as previously expressed or exhibited, would be, we may arrive at a different conclusion. If it is more convincingly established that the patient would indeed have wanted to forgo treatment with antibiotics, then the principle of autonomy could be invoked in future decisions about their use. Also, as the course of the disease continues, (1) the avoidance-of-harm principle would lead to increasing skepticism that prolonging treatment confers more benefits than harm and (2) the ever-increasing drain on the family's and society's resources would turn the consideration-of-others'-interest principle toward support for withholding treatment. Accordingly, we might well end up withholding the use of antibiotics in the future.

Case 3: The Cancer Patient

This patient is very assertive in wanting to direct drug treatment —requesting (a) laetrile rather than chemotherapy, (b) a pain-killing drug in dosages perhaps sufficient to hasten death, and (c) heroin as the pain-killing drug.

Laetrile

Regarding the demand to take laetrile rather than chemotherapy, the autonomy issue turns upon the reasonableness of the patient's informed deliberation and assessment of best interest. In this case, the prognosis is crucial in judging reasonableness. The physicians could argue that chemotherapy, rather than the worthless drug laetrile, is the reasonable choice after informed deliberation and consideration of the patient's best interests, only if the chemotherapy treatment had a decent chance of curing the cancer. But the patient probably has at most six months to live, even with chemotherapy; so this argument falters. No matter how much one regards the laetrile treatment to be a waste of time, the fact remains that chemotherapy offers no higher prospects of success. Physicians should make sure that the patient fully understands the medical profession's evaluation of laetrile. But given this desperate a situation, we cannot deny the patient's autonomy on the grounds that the laetrile demand is unreasonable. A similar analysis occurs with the avoidance of harm principle. Given the patient's prognosis, one has a difficult time showing that laetrile causes harm.

The chief objections to use of laetrile arise when we consider others' interests. Society has an interest in limiting use of any worthless drug that fosters false hopes in others. Physicians have an obligation to use the current state of knowledge to provide effective, rather than worthless, treatments to their patients. We could probably satisfy society's interest here by requiring that laetrile only be given to terminal patients and by publicizing this requirement widely. The physicians' obligation, however, cannot be accommodated so simply. To compel, or even ask, a physician to prescribe a worthless drug attacks the essence of what it means to be a physician. For medicine as a profession to maintain self-respect and retain public trust, it cannot sanction worthless treatments—no matter what other reasons may justify them. Moreover, given the importance of medicine to human life, the physicians' obligation takes precedence over an individual patient's autonomous choice to take laetrile. This judgment holds for now, even though we grant a possibility, however unlikely, that laetrile may prove itself to be effective in treating cancer at some time in the future.

Physicians should not prescribe laetrile, even if a terminal patient demands it. Some allowances, of course, can be made for carefully controlled experimental uses. Perhaps, in deference to the principles of autonomy and avoidance of harm, laetrile may even justifiably be made available to the aged and dying in some circumstances. But professionals in medicine should not be the ones prescribing it.

Dosages Sufficient to Hasten Death

Given the analysis for the patient with multiple sclerosis, there is good reason to grant an autonomous request for a pain-killing drug in dosages that may also hasten death. If anything, the cancer patient's case is stronger because the life-expectancy is shorter and the pain involved seems to be more sharply determinable by others. That is to say, the multiple sclerosis patient's misery probably depends more upon self-evaluation than the cancer patient's pain (although granting this does not establish that she suffers less pain.)

But there is another, independent argument to consider. One can appeal to the principle of double effect—arguing that a drug dosage *sufficient to alleviate pain* is the effect intended and any hastening of death that happens to occur is an unintended second effect. Moreover, one can argue that the intended good effect is at least equal in worth to the unintended second effect. The justification would appeal to the same points made in discussing avoidance of harm, sanctity of life, and acceptance of death in the case of the multiple sclerosis patient: (1) Alleviation of pain avoids harm here in a situation in which death can no longer be looked upon as an ultimate harm; (2) respect for the sanctity of life here does not require that we only take measures that prolong life; and (3) there is a need for accepting death in this situation. If we combine the patient's autonomous request with this independent argument, we conclude that drug dosages sufficient to control pain should be given even if doing so hastens death. We need to establish, or course, that alleviation of pain is the real intention in administering the drug.

Heroin

The patient's request for heroin as a pain-killer differs fundamentally from the laetrile demand in that heroin is not regarded to be a worthless drug by the medical profession. It is quite effective in alleviating pain, which is a primary goal of medical treatment for this dying cancer patient. So why is there a problem? Basically, there are three sorts of problems: (1) It is alleged that heroin is risky or hastens death by depressing respiration and by requiring ever larger doses to counteract the rapidly increasing tolerance of the drug by the patient; (2) it is alleged that heroin produces addiction and euphoria in a way that reduces the patient to a suspended state of "living death" unworthy of a human being; and (3) it is alleged, in the United States at least, that storing of heroin for patient use is an invitation to theft, given the considerable number of crimes related to drug addiction. Opponents argue that there are enough alternative drugs available to control pain without using heroin and encountering its attendant problems. The allegations point to problems associated with autonomy, avoidance of harm, sanctity of life, and others' interests. These allegations, however, do not go unchallenged. For example, it has been pointed out that any heroin stored in hospices and hospital pharmacies in the US would amount to only a small percentage (less than 5%) of the total amount of heroin available in the country illegally. The British hospice movement provides the stiffest denials of allegations (1) and (2). British physicians report that heroin, when carefully given after detailed assessment of the patient's condition, (a) does not depress respiration, (b) does not run into the difficulties of increased tolerance, (c) does not produce euphoria, (d) allows the patient to live in a relatively normal way, and (e) creates no problem of addiction that causes concern. Moreover, if there is any hastening of death, this is an unintended secondary effect, the primary intended effect being the alleviation of pain. Supporters of heroin use for terminal cancer patients argue that it has many advantages as a pain reliever—such as lack of nausea, greater potency, and quick absorption and relief of pain. Some supporters of the British hospice movement also argue that effective pain control—including use of heroin when necessary—is the key to eliminating the need for "mercy killing": If patients can be assured that their pain will be controlled, they will not want drastic measures taken to end their lives.

What should we say here about this patient's request for heroin as a pain reliever?

Regarding allegation (1), we face a problem because of the factual dispute involved. Rather than trying to settle this, suppose, for our purposes, we just assume that prescribed doses of heroin might in some way hasten death. We then can apply the analysis already given to handle this possibility.

The British experience with use of heroin in hospices tends strongly to refute allegation (2). The fears about euphoria, degrading addiction, and a "living death" seem to be unfounded. Accordingly, any associated concerns regarding loss of autonomy, causing harm to patients, and not respecting the sanctity of life are not convincing.

Allegation (3) requires consideration of others' interests. Any benefits of allowing heroin use to control pain should be weighed against potential costs because of any greater likelihood of theft of heroin supplies arising from drug addiction problems. Although any heroin needed for hospices and hospital pharmacies might be small relative to other sources of heroin available, criminals might see these places as "easy targets" for supplies—thereby requiring a disruptive amount of security protection in the hospices and hospital pharmacies. Although this potential cost is a legitimate concern, it is no greater than what we put up with when we provide protection in other situations—e.g., for victims of threats, for radioactive substances, and for materials in laboratories. Accordingly, this concern does not outweigh the earlier considerations that support use of heroin. We might want to qualify this conclusion somewhat. If it can be shown that drugs other than heroin are just as effective in controlling pain, then there is no need to incur the added cost of providing greater security protection for places that store heroin. At this point, however the burden of proof lies with those who claim that these alternative drugs are available.

Case 4: The Organic Brain Syndrome Patient

This patient's periods of confusion, paranoia, and decreased intellectual function create problems in the present, with the likelihood of greater problems in the future. (We are assuming that the dementia is irreversible.) If the patient has such a poor prognosis and is difficult to handle, is it acceptable to administer highly sedating drugs, such as barbiturates, to maintain control and ease the staff's burden?

At first glance, anyone not responsible for this patient's care will probably judge this alternative to be terrible. It seems to violate almost all the ethical principles we are working with. It further decreases whatever autonomy the patient had left and thus causes harm; it violates the sanctity of life by treating the patient as a thing to be manipulated for the benefit of the staff; and it sets a bad precedent for solving problems in a society.

Suppose that some staff members see this differently, however. They see little point in protecting an autonomy that barely exists and putting up with a troublesome patient, besides. The heavy sedation is a small sacrifice for the patient to make (perhaps not even felt to be a sacrifice)—especially since the patient has no hope of getting back to normal and the patient's condition will continue to deteriorate. Are these considerations sufficient to change the initial judgment?

Suppose that we accept the legitimacy of these considerations and think about the situation of the patient now placed under heavy sedation. The patient now subsists in a semi-coma, much like a "living death." Consequently, the patient's treatment status changes. Care will turn more toward making the patient comfortable and perhaps even accepting approaches that hasten death—such as withholding antibiotics. What is troubling, even reprehensible, here is the way this patient's changed status is medically induced—through prescription of a heavy sedative. The prescribed drug seriously violates the avoidance of harm principle by making the patient's condition worse. Accordingly, we are left again with the conclusion that heavy sedation is unacceptable. So a milder drug should be used.

Rules for Prescribing Drugs

We can summarize the direction of this analysis by formulating the following rules in prescribing drugs for the aged and dying:

1. Physicians should not prescribed drugs known to be worthless.
2. Physicians should not prescribe, or withdraw, previously pre-

scribed drugs when doing so is likely to cause some new medical problem for the patient.

3. Physicians should respect patient autonomy in making decisions about prescription drugs.

   a. Drugs that reduce patient autonomy should be avoided as much as possible.

   b. Given an autonomous request by the aged and dying, with holding of drugs such as antibiotics and even use of life-ending drugs in some instances is not beyond the range of what is morally acceptable.

   c. Faced with a terminal disease with little life-expectancy, the aged and dying when acting autonomously should not be pre vented from taking even drugs judged to be worthless by the medical profession.

4. Patients insisting upon maintaining autonomy in making requests about drug treatment should take as much responsibility as possible in the administering of any drug. For example, if the request for a lethal injection is morally acceptable, preferably, patients should administer it themselves (under appropriate medical conditions).

5. Physicians should be allowed to refuse to prescribe or administer death-hastening drugs when their aged or dying patients, acting autonomously, request them—although they are obligated to transfer patients to other physicians in such cases.

6. When patients' wishes about drug treatment are unknown or the patient clearly wanted life-preserving treatment, then life-preserving drugs should not be withheld or life-ending drugs administered—unless, over time, the patient's condition has deteriorated sufficiently to suggest reconsideration of the previous decision in terms of avoidance of harm, acceptance of death, and others' interests.

7. Sufficient drug dosages should be prescribed to control pain in terminal patients, even if the dosages themselves hasten death.

8. Heroin should be allowed as a pain killing drug for the aged and dying—unless it can be shown that alternative drugs are equally effective in controlling pain.

Specific conditions, of course, are relevant to any decision. We need accurate information about the patient's condition, about whether or not patients' decisions satisfy the standards for autonomy, about the precise circumstances of patients' pain, and about the real intentions of any proposed treatment. But the formulated rules should prove useful as well. It is hoped that they are reasonable enough to provide guidance in this sensitive, important area.

Selected and Annotated Bibliography

The best general source for recent work on ethical issues associated with prescribing drugs is Le Roy Walters and Tamar Joy Kahn, *Bibliography of Bioethics* (Washington: Kennedy Institute of Ethics, issued annually). Government Regulation/Drugs and Patient Care/Drugs are the relevant subject headings.

General Medical Background

See Kenneth A. Conrad and Rubin Bressler, eds., *Drug Therapy for the Elderly* (St. Louis: C.V. Mosby Co.; 1982), especially Chs. 12–15. Also, see Richard H. Davis and William K. Smith, eds., *Drugs and the Elderly* (Los Angeles: University of Southern California Press, 1975), especially Eric Pfeiffer's "Use of Drugs Which Influence Behavior in the Elderly: Promises, Pitfalls and Perspectives." For a brief account of various diseases of the elderly, I turned to Mary W. Falconer, Michael V. Altamura, and Helen Duncan Behnke, *Aging Patients: A Guide for Their Care* (New York: Springer Publishing Co., 1976).

Ethical Background

An extended, very valuable discussion of relevant ethical principles can be found in Tom L. Beauchamp and James F. Childress, *Principles of Biomedical Ethics* (New York: Oxford University Press, 1983), 2nd ed. A discussion of autonomy and some other important issues can be found in David H. Smith, ed., *Respect and*

Care in Medical Ethics (Lanham, Maryland: University Press of America, 1984). Anne Donchin's "Personal Autonomy, Life Plans, and Chronic Illness" in this volume is especially interesting. For a legal perspective, see P.D.G. Skegg, *Law, Ethics, and Medicine: Studies in Medical Law* (Oxford: Clarendon Press, 1984)— although one has to expect some legalistic terminology. The book contains a pertinent chapter, "Drugs Hastening Death." For an anthology dealing with the issue of death and dying, see Michael D. Bayles and Dallas M. High, eds., *Medical Treatment of the Dying: Moral Issues* (Cambridge: Schenkman Publishing Co., 1978).

Drugs and Pain Control

See the *Bibliography of Bioethics, op. cit.*, for various articles dealing with disputes regarding use of laetrile or heroin. For an overview of the laetrile issue, see Gerald E. Markle and James C. Petersen, eds., *Politics, Science, and Cancer: The Laetrile Phenomenon* (Boulder: Westview Press, 1980). For background on use of morphine and heroin in treating pain, see R.G. Twycross, "Ethical and Clinical Aspects of Pain Treatment in Cancer Patients," *Acta Anaesthesiologica Scandinavica*, supplement 74, vol. 26, 1982, pp. 83–90. Also, see K.M. Foley, "Clinical Assessment of Cancer Pain," in the same supplement, pp. 91–96.

Animals as a Source of
Human Transplant Organs

Introduction

In "The Rights and Wrongs of Animal Use for Human Organ Transplant," Richard Werner asks his readers to consider a situation in which a superior race of extraterrestrial beings (the Bios) lands on Earth. Physically, Bios are much like humans, and these beings want to harvest human organs for the purpose of saving Bio lives. The Bios agree not to take human organs for transplant unless human beings can be convinced of the rightness of such action by rational argument; hence, a context for discussion is set in which readers will side, not with those who desire to kill to use others' organs, but rather with those who will be killed for the purpose of organ transplant.

In the course of the human–Bio debate concerning the propriety of harvesting human organs, three moral positions serve as foci for discussion. First, Werner considers natural law arguments against the use of human organs for Bio transplant. Werner rejects natural law theory, and argues that the position leads to speciesism and an unjustified bias for the status quo. Next, Werner considers utilitarian arguments against the harvesting of human organs for use by Bios. In rejecting this view, Werner argues that it is biased in favor of sentient creatures, and should be rejected for the same reasons that we reject racism, sexism, and speciesism. Finally, Werner considers the moral position defended by his fictional Bios. In this view, all life is worthy of respect; however, not all living things are due the same degree of moral consideration. How much moral consideration a living thing is due depends upon the entity's capacities and abilities. The more capacities and abilities a thing has, the more worthy it is of moral consideration; beings worthy of the highest degree of moral consideration are called "persons."

The Bios claim that although persons have a moral obligation to produce minimum damage to other forms of life, they also have a right to take what is necessary for the satisfaction of their own basic needs. Because Bios need human organs for their survival, they argue that they have a right to harvest such organs, at least the organs of humans who do not possess those abilities and capacities necessary for qualifying them as persons, e.g., unwanted babies, abortuses, and mental defectives.

If Werner's "Bio argument" is correct, it is morally permissible for persons to use animal organs for transplantation purposes, but it is also morally permissible for persons to harvest the organs of human nonpersons for life saving purposes. In "Animal Parts, Human Wholes: On the Use of Animals as a Source of Organs For Human Transplants," R. G. Frey arrives at essentially the same conclusion; however, Frey's essay differs from Werner's in at least two significant ways. First, whereas Werner rejects utilitarianism as being unjustifiably biased in favor of sentient creatures, Frey embraces utilitarianism. Thus, Frey's analysis shows that acceptance of utilitarianism does not require that one be opposed to the use of animal organs for human transplant. Second, Frey points out that xenografts (transplantations of organs or tissues from a member of one species to a member of another) are less likely to succeed than transplantations that occur between different members of the same species. Hence, for transplantation purposes, there is better reason to prefer the use of organs taken from human nonpersons, e.g., severely retarded infants, than organs taken from nonhuman animals.

In "Animals As a Source of Human Transplant Organs," James L. Nelson surveys a number of arguments that have been used in opposition to, and support of, use of animals for human benefit. After surveying these arguments, Nelson concludes that considerations of impartial moral reason make the use of animal organs for human transplant morally problematic. Still, Nelson claims that the issue cannot be said to be fully settled, for the decision to use animal organs for human transplant need not be made solely on the basis of "impartial moral reason." Indeed, Nelson argues that parents' partiality for their children is a virtue, and that this virtue may, in some circumstances, impose a moral obligation upon parents to seek animal organs for use in prolonging their children's lives. In cases such as this, parents are caught in a moral dilemma: Considerations of impartial moral reason indicate that they should not use animal organs to prolong their children's lives, while parental concern demands that they attempt to secure animal organs for transplantation. When faced with such a dilemma, Nelson argues that it would be morally proper for parents to seek animal organs, because this course of action allows parents to keep faith with more morally relevant circumstances than the alternate course of action.

The Rights and Wrongs of Animal Use for Human Organ Transplant

Richard Werner

What follows are the remains of a diary believed to have been written by Dr. Fran Quinn, a human scientist, immediately before the Great Transformation of 2037.

July 7th: The Bios have landed! After two years of radio communication we have finally made physical contact. Our first encounter with an alien life form and I'm on the inside! My God, they are so much like us: almost identical biology, and rational featherless bipeds to boot! Yet they are different too. Their telepathic communication seems so eerie; it is as if they read our thoughts at will and only allow us to understand those of their thoughts they want. And their technology and intelligence! It is so advanced from our own. I almost want to say it is totally different because of their different history and seemingly advanced conceptual capacities. Intellectually, conceptually, technologically they stand to us as we do to the other animals. I hope they remain friendly, although if they don't there is little we can do at this point.

July 9th: The Bios are so kind, so wonderful. The Bios remind me of stories of St. Francis or Ghandi, perhaps even of Jesus. They care so much about one another, yet also about all other life forms, including us humans. They seem to appreciate each entity for what it is, as well as for what it will become. They are so in touch with life and the universe around them, something we humans rarely seem to sense, if at all. Compared to the Bios, it is as though we don't really *care* about the life around us, about the universe itself. They seem to experience and understand on a deeper level. It is as though we only see the shadows of things, while they see reality for what it is. They remind me of Plato's allegory of the cave. There is little chance that they will bring anything but good for humanity.

July 22nd: I can't believe it! How can they do this to us! After appearing so kind, so caring, so superior, now they want to *use* us like we are nothing but spare parts. The only reason they have made contact is because of our amazingly similar biology and the fact that they can use our organs for transplant into their own bodies, thereby saving the lives of dying Bios. Organ transplant! That is to be the price we pay for accepting the benefits of their care and technology. Strip-mining us for organs!

Is this to become the purpose, the telos of human existence? Just who do they think they are to do this to us? After all, we are human beings with natural rights and human dignity. Don't they see that we deserve to be respected as humans? We are not mere animals whose only concern is pleasure and pain. We have hopes and plans and dreams that their domination will only frustrate. Our freedom is essential to our being, and our liberation from their power will become necessary if we are to continue to exist as people. We are more than mere organ-producing machines; we are beings with autonomous wills that desire more than mere physical pleasure and security. Why can't they see? Is their superior intelligence clouded by their own selfish interests?

Can't they see that we are the end product of our planet's evolution; that we are the crown of earthly creation? HUMAN BEINGS WITH NATURAL RIGHTS; that is what we are. What the Bios are proposing to do to us is a perversion of the natural order of things. We have the *natural* right to use nature for our ends and purposes. But as human beings, it is wrong to *use* us in the same way. Our biology, our evolution has made us special and given us dominion over the earth. Even the *Bible* tells us that human beings have dominion over the earth. What the Bios want is to destroy that natural order, to interrupt the process of both biological and social evolution. It is unnatural and, hence, it goes without saying that it is wrong. Why can't they understand that? Has their power simply gone to their heads?

Or is it that they fail to understand because they are not part of the natural order of this planet? Their world is different from ours. A different evolution, different climate, just plain different. Because they are not part of the natural order of earth, they can never understand how perverse, how unnatural, it is for them to use us as they plan. By their lights, in terms of their natural history, it may be right, but here on earth it is simply wrong and unnatural.

July 27th: The Bios' arguments seem so rational. They are so compelling when I listen to their telepathic communication that I begin to suspect that they are playing games with my mind. Perhaps by writing down their arguments I will later read what I have written and be able to see the flaws in their reasoning when I am unhampered by their telepathic interference.

Nevertheless, they are surely right about one thing. The very notion of what is natural and unnatural is itself ambiguous and relative. According to one sense of "natural," everything we've done since we left the hunting/gathering stage of human history has been unnatural—everything from indoor plumbing, to medicine, to farming. On the other hand, everything we do and create is natural since it is the product of social creatures with a social history—everything from the wars and atrocities, to the stress of postindustrial life, to underarm deodorants. According to these two senses of what is natural, either almost everything we do and how we do it is unnatural and wrong, or almost everything we do is natural and right. The former sense of "natural" is too narrow, whereas the latter is too broad.

Yet a third sense of the natural would have it that the natural is the norm. Whatever most people do is natural and right, whereas the activities of the few are unnatural and wrong. If most people do not practice oral sex, or cremation, or vegetarianism, then these activities are unnatural and wrong. If most people eat Hostess Twinkies, use hair mousse, and bottle-feed their babies, then these activities are natural and right. Such statistical norms have proven to be highly variable both historically and culturally. But the natural is supposedly fixed by nature, unchanging, nonaccidental. If nothing else, the endless variety of what is "normal" shows that the norm has little to do with what is natural. The third sense merely confuses what is natural with what is ordinary. Clearly, as the Bios put it, such uses of the word "natural" are merely disguised ways of sanctioning the status quo. Such uses confuse nature with nurture.

Further, the Bios argue, there is a confusion here between what is natural and what is right or good or desirable. Death, disease, and acne are natural, yet few among us have them high on our list of what is right or good or desirable. Antibiotics, long underwear, and such technological cocoons as cars, airplanes, and modern office buildings are unnatural, yet few among us condemn them as wrong and immoral. Just as we use the word "natural" ambiguously, there is confusion at work when we attempt to treat everything that is natural as good or right and everything that is unnatural as bad or wrong. The ambiguity of the word "natural" allows us deceptively, and sometimes persuasively, to define it to condone and condemn morally whatever we may approve or disapprove emotively.

July 28th: This Singer guy is terrific! And Feinberg is wonderful! Together they're a match for the Bios. Their arguments are as persuasive as the Bios'.[1]

I can see in my entry of July 22nd another mistake in my thinking. Being human is simply being a member of a certain biological category; it is a biological fact about us. But humans as members of a certain biological category have no special moral worth. Biological categories do not assign moral worth. Biological facts, by themselves, do not entail moral prescriptions. To think that humans are morally superior simply because of their biology is to commit the same kind of mistake the racist, nationalist, sexist, or classist commits. It is to think that one's own group is special, morally more worthy, just because it is one's own group. Human history abounds with such ethnocentrism. Our anthropocentrism commits the same logical and moral mistake.

All of the characteristics that we think make us special creatures, our self-consciousness, our use of language, our use of tools and technology, our moral sensibilities, are, arguably, shared with other creatures on this planet. We consider ourselves to be persons, to be rational, valuing beings who are autonomous centers of conscious life. Yet it is arguable that apes, whales, and dolphins have all of these attributes; and we misuse them just as the Bios plan to do to us. If characteristics such as self-consciousness, language use, tool use, moral sensibilities, autonomy, rationality make an entity a member of the moral community, then apes, whales, and dolphins have as just a claim as do we.

These animals are not only conscious centers of experience capable of feeling pleasure and pain, it is also reasonable to believe that they are self-conscious beings capable of planning and carrying out their plans. They do so consciously, willfully, and not merely instinctively as do the other animals. They appear to be as autonomous as we, albeit *perhaps* not as intelligent. But intelligence has never been the mark of moral standing; if it were we would award people rights on the basis of their IQ rather than on the basis of their personhood. Singer and Feinberg admit that the Bios are right to say that we have treated these other animals far worse than the Bios plan to treat us. Not only do we use apes for organ transplants, we run scientific and medical experiments on them. Many of these experiments are cruel and dangerous for the animals; all are demeaning. We eat whales and dolphins. We train all of these animals. We constantly use them as mere means to our own ends. We show them no respect.

Apes have even been taught to communicate with us, although some scholars argue that they don't really use language, they only manipulate symbols. But how is that different from human babies or mental defectives or, for that matter, from any human? Where do we draw the line on language and self-consciousness in a nondeceptive, unselfish way? Why do we think that our species is so different, so much more special than all other life forms on this planet? If we are all the products of a common evolution, it would be bizarre in the extreme for homo sapiens to stand out so sharply, so distinctly.

Yet Singer and Feinberg are correct. Just because we have mistreated these animals in the past does not justify the Bios in mistreating us. We humans have evolved beyond thinking that an eye for an eye is just punishment, or that two wrongs can make a right. We should mend our ways with respect to the higher mammals like apes, whales, and dolphins, those that qualify as persons, and the Bios should leave us alone.

Even if we are the only naturally occurring persons on this planet, the distinction between persons and human beings is an important one. The existence of the Bios proves the point. They are not human beings; they are not members of our species; yet they are persons in every sense of the word. When people believe in God, or the devil, or in angels they are distinguishing between persons and human beings. God is certainly not human, but God is a person on most accounts. Likewise for the devil and angels. We make the distinction every time we watch a cartoon on TV populated with rabbits, pigs, ducks, mice, and cats, all of whom we understand to be persons but not human beings. Conceptually, we are and have been committed to the distinction between human beings and persons for a long time.

Personhood, that is the key to this whole mess. Lower life forms, such as insects, plants, and protozoa, are not due moral consideration, for they are not conscious; they lack sentiency. They cannot have interests because they lack the conceptual capacity to form interests. Hence, they cannot be harmed. But any creature that suffers is due moral consideration. So sentiency or consciousness gets an animal into the realm of the moral community. But *self*-consciousness, the ability to have self-designed preferences or goals, what philosophers call "an autonomous will," is a step above mere consciousness within the moral community.

Self-conscious beings are rational, valuing, autonomous centers of conscious life. Self-conscious beings are truly PERSONS; merely conscious beings are just animals. Self-conscious beings are harmed not only by physical pain, but also suffer mental anguish when their rational will is frustrated. Because they can conceptualize their own future, they fear death. As such, persons have a far greater capacity for pain and suffering, pleasure and happiness as a result of their self-conscious abilities. Because they can have hopes and dreams and plans, because they have values, because they are rational and autonomous, they can be made to suffer in different ways—both qualitatively and quantitatively different ways.

Accordingly, there is a hierarchy within the moral community. Self-conscious beings have a right to life because they have rational preferences or goals that can be frustrated. They have a rational interest in remaining alive. They desire to live out a normal life. Merely conscious animals may be due moral consideration because they can suffer physical pain and may have an interest in preventing suffering, but they lack the wherewithal to have truly *rational* preferences or goals. They don't have a formed *interest* in remaining alive because they can't even understand what "remaining alive" or "dying" would mean. They don't make plans or set goals, except instinctively. Have you ever seen a mere animal with a social calendar or a grocery list? They don't even lament or fear their own death.

We can only harm a mere animal if we cause it physical pain or frustrate its instincts. There is no other way to violate its interests. Killing it quickly and painlessly does not cause it physical pain or frustrate its instincts.[2] So we can kill mere animals as long as we do it quickly and painlessly, since killing them does not harm them or their interest. Simply put, mere animals don't have a moral right to life, whereas persons do. Even though it is permissible to kill painlessly a mere animal to use its organs to preserve the life of a person, it is wrong to kill one person to provide organs for another. That's why what the Bios want to do to us is so wrong. Persons really do have dominion over the mere animals.

Animals with self-consciousness like apes and whales and dolphins do have rights and ought not to be used as we have done.

Singer and Feinberg are right about that. Like us, they are persons, and we have committed an egregious wrong by exploiting these animals. We shouldn't even use such nonhuman persons for organ transplants, let alone experiment upon or eat them, since they have a fully fledged right to life. We have also been wrong in how we have raised and slaughtered most mere animals for food and fun, since our practices entail unnecessary pain and suffering for the dumb animals. We must stop these practices.

But, again, the issue is deeper than first appears. As Singer and Feinberg argue, we must distinguish between normal adult members of a species that produces persons—those who have a developed capacity for personhood—and defectives and infant members who are not persons—those who, at best, have the capacity for personhood. Those who are not yet persons may be killed painlessly to serve the needs of persons as long as no other person has an interest in the nonperson human.[3]

A potential person has, at best, potential rights. A fully developed person has actual rights. An actual right to life would take precedence over a potential right to life. Just consider what a 15-year-old's potential right to drink is worth in a bar, or what his or her potential right to vote is worth on election day. So organ transplant from a baby baboon into a baby human, to save the latter's life, would be justified, if the killing of the baboon was painless and other adult baboons were not negatively affected.

Moreover, like the word "natural," the word "potential" is highly ambiguous and greatly misued. In the world of modern physics, anything is potentially anything else. In theory, all we need do is rearrange its atomic or subatomic structure. So any object that is large enough is a potential person, even a bag of toenails, a truck, or a large rock.[4]

Then there are human gametes. Each sperm and ovum is potentially a person. If we are to count potential rights as the equal of actual rights, then each gamete has the right to be conceived and developed into an actual person.

Unless we want to grant fully fledged moral rights to toenails, trucks, gametes, and all of the rest of the furniture of the earth, it would seem that the fact that a baby baboon is a potential person is irrelevant, at least for the issue of organ transplant.

August 1st: The Bios persist in pushing the arguments. They claim that they won't use us for organ transplants if they can't convince us that they are rationally justified in so doing. That, they say, is respecting us fully as autonomous persons, as *rational*, autonomous persons. Perhaps they are right, but I must admit that I still find their arguments highly persuasive, and that worries me. Is it their arguments that convince me or some subtle form of mind control caused by their telepathic powers?

The Bios' position is rather complex, although not complicated. It rests on several distinctions.[5] An activity or event is "good for an entity" only when it promotes or protects the entity's good. To "promote or protect an entity's good" is either to bring about a state of affairs not yet realized in its existence that is conducive to its well-being or to get rid of a condition in its existence that is detrimental to its well-being.

An entity has a "good of its own" the Bios claim, only when it makes sense to speak of what is good or bad *for* the entity in question, and without reference to any other entity. According to this definition, each living creature would have a good of its own tied to the fact that it is a teleological center of life. We can speak meaningfully of what is good or bad for a baby, a horse, a worm, a fly, a tomato plant, or even a protozoan. But it makes little sense to speak of what is good or bad for a brick, a pile of sand, or a bucket of water. Human artifacts may seem to have a good of their own (e.g., a car, a piano, or a computer), but this is only because their human creators invested them with purpose for humans. Hence, we need to make reference to other entities (i.e., humans) to explain what is good and bad for human artifacts, and, accordingly, they do not have a good of their own.

Here the Bios' position diverges sharply from the positions of Singer and Feinberg. Although the latter two delimit the moral community to sentient beings, the Bios expand the moral community to include all life. The difference centers around the notion of "having an interest." According to the Bios and contrary to Singer and Feinberg, "having (forming) interests" may be sufficient for a being to have a good of its own, but it is not necessary. Hence, the Bios argue that having (forming) interests is not a necessary condition for a being to have a good of its own.

A being's formed interests may or may not coincide with that being's actual interests, the Bios argue. Obviously, we are sometimes mistaken about our own interests. This would be impossible if formed or perceived interests coincided with actual interests. Further, it is the being's actual interests that are relevant to the being's own good and, one would think, whether it is due moral consideration. Promoting or protecting the being's good would, it would seem, turn on the being's actual interests rather than its formed or perceived interests. Thus, in terms of moral consideration, a being's *actual* interests rather than its formed or perceived interests is what is relevant.

In addition, it would seem to be irrelevant from the moral point of view whether or not the being can form or have perceived interests. What is relevant is whether the being has actual interests, whether it can be said to have a good of its own. Consequently the Bios argue that any entity that can be benefited or harmed directly has a good of its own, regardless of whether it has formed or perceived interests. All plants and simpler animal life appear to lack consciousness or the ability to make choices among alternatives confronting them. They lack formed or perceived interests. Yet we can still benefit or harm them, promote or harm their actual interests. Similarly, a whole biotic community can have actual interests and, thereby, a good of its own. Even the biosphere of the earth has actual interests that can be advanced or retarded according to the Bios' distinction.

The Bios also argue that a creature's good of its own is distinct from its "inherent worth." One can acknowledge that a creature has a good of its own, yet ask, "why should I care about the creature or its well-being?" Indeed, the Bios think that we humans constantly engage in such thought and behavior. A creature has inherent worth, the Bios argue, just in case the entity *deserves* moral concern and consideration as an end in itself and for its own sake. As such, all persons have a duty, no matter how small that duty may be, to promote or protect the entity's good.

But how do we determine whether a creature has inherent worth? The Bios claim that such questions can only be addressed meaningfully to persons, to rational, valuing beings who are autonomous centers of conscious life. They are the only beings capable of understanding and responding meaningfully to such questions. Furthermore, the Bios argue, each person has inherent worth because this is the only way we can make sense of our own personhood. Solely by virtue of the fact that I am a center of autonomous choice and valuation and, thereby, give direction to my life on the basis of my own values, I have an actual interest in ensuring that others respect my autonomous choices based on my values. So, by parity of reason, by the logical rule that similar cases are to be judged similarly, I must be willing to grant a similar entitlement to all other persons. The only way in which one can make sense of this while living among a community of persons is to adopt what the Bios call the attitude of respect for persons:

> "Each person should give equal weight to every person's value-system and at the same time make it possible for each to pursue the realization of his or her own value-system in ways compatible with everyone else's similar pursuit."[6]

The attitude of respect for persons is just the realization that persons have inherent worth as persons and also an acknowledgment of what that worth entails.

But once we acknowledge the attitude of respect for persons, that persons have inherent worth, we are also committed to acknowledging the inherent worth of all living creatures and biotic communities, of any entity with a good its own. As a creature, I have an actual interest in my own inherent worth, of my own good as a creature. I have the actual interest whether or not I have a formed perceived interest in my own inherent worth. Parity of reason, the logical rule that similar cases are to be judged similarly, commits me to respect other entities' good of their own in terms of which they can be helped or harmed, commits me to acknowledge that they have an actual interest in their own inherent worth, which deserves protection and promotion.

The attitude of respect for life follows from the fact that all of us have an actual interest in the promotion and protection of our inherent worth, in the same manner that the attitude of respect for persons follows from the fact that all persons have an actual interest in the promotion and protection of their personhood. The attitude of respect for life is just the realization that each life has inherent worth and an acknowledgment of what that worth entails.[7] Finally, the attitude of respect for life leads us to the attitude of respect for nature since each biosphere, including the biosphere of the earth, has a good of its own and, thereby, has inherent worth deserving of our respect.

It will not do to argue that respect for life should be delimited to those with the conceptual capacity to return the favor (i.e., persons). The point does not rest on a mythological social contract or some prudential notion of *quid pro quo* but on the logical rule of parity of reason and an accurate assessment of what is morally relevant and what are our actual interests. All of us think that our own good as a creature is worthy of pursuit, that our own life and whatever is conducive to it is valuable, whereas what truly harms us and is harmful to our life is bad and worthy of avoidance. All of us have an actual interest in the promotion and protection of our own good as a creature—whether or not it is a formed or perceived interest.

To attempt to delimit such actual interests to persons or to humans is no different from the racist or sexist or classist who would delimit them only to white folks, or men, or those with proper birth or wealth. Such stipulations are surely morally arbitrary since each and every life has an actual interest in its own good as a creature, and it is our own good as a creature that we have an actual interest in protecting and promoting. If we count the protection and promotion of our own good as morally relevant, then reason tells us that we should count as morally relevant the protection and promotion of the good of any creature or biosphere. A good is a good, no matter whose good it may be. A harm is a harm, no matter whose harm it may be. Likewise, a life is a life, no matter whose life it may be. Hence, parity of reason should commit us to the attitude of respect for life, of acknowledging that each living creature as well as each biotic community has inherent worth, a good of its own that is worthy of our protection and promotion.

It is because of a deep respect for life, the Bios argue, that they care so much about the creatures and things around them, that they see the world differently from us, and, as a result, move and act in the world with greater grace.[8] Because we deny the attitude of respect for life and, at best and only rarely, adopt merely the attitude of respect for persons, are we so much less aware and appreciate so much less of the world around us. We simply don't *care* about the *world*, the way that they do. Our self and our things, rather than the beauty and well-being of the earth's biosphere, are our primary concern in life, our fundamental project. As a result, we can't see the world or live in the world as the Bios.

We do not see the world as filled with beings of value and inherent worth, as a world of wonder; we see it as something to be used and manipulated according to our perceived interests. Too frequently, our perceived interests are contrary to the actual interests of the rest of the biosphere in which we live and our own actual interests as a species.[9] We simply see *things*, ignoring the relationships among them. Further, we only see things in terms of what use they are to us rather than in terms of their own inherent worth. Just think of our recent predilection for the cost/benefit analysis of social problems, including environmental problems. Cost and benefit for whom? "Of what *use* is it?" is one of our favorite rhetorical questions. We ask the question not only of events and things, but increasingly of other life forms and even of one another.

We can only see what we know. Our inability to see the world of the Bios is caused by the metaphysics imbedded within our culture. This embeddedness is the historical consequence of the success of technology coupled with the identification of technology with the scientific worldview of such thinkers as Descartes, Galileo, and Hobbes. Like these philosophers, we understand the universe as composed of lifeless, valueless matter that acts only according to the laws of physics. We see ourselves as selfish maximizers of pleasure who are subject to the same laws of physics, as well as to the laws of economics. Nature is an infinite storehouse to be plundered for our enjoyment. Our acceptance of this worldview makes us into machine-like aliens in our actual biological environment. We are estranged from our actual life-world and that which gives meaning to our existence. Our worldview serves as a self-fulfilling prophecy for what we have become, what we are. Our worldview renders us incapable of seeing and understanding the beauty and value of the universe in which we live, of seeing what is there plainly to be seen. Instead, we trade meaning for pleasure, purpose for power, and life for consumption.

No wonder our present century, like no other before it, screams of human atrocity after human atrocity while it proclaims itself the pinnacle of civilization and civility. No wonder the human condition is likened to a homesickness. No wonder we seek to dominate not only our environment, but one another. We estrange ourselves from everything that is conceivably meaningful in our world. We are out of touch with any meaningful reality. Our own anthropocentrism destroyed the value and meaning of the world around us. We forget how to care not only about the world, but about each other, and even about our own selves.

Our lack of care about nature leads, naturally enough, to our lack of care about one another, since humans are merely a part of nature. In turn, our lack of care about other humans leads to a lack of care about our selves, since each of us is just another human. Our lack of care reflects on itself; it becomes reflexive. All subjects are reduced to mere objects, all life to mere things. Our lack of care rapidly translates into a need to dominate and control first nature, then other people, and finally our selves in a fruitless attempt to fill the emptiness in our lives with more things. How else would a selfish maximizer of pleasure go forth into the world? We are uncaring, alienated beings out of touch with nature, other people, and ourselves, while our fundamental project is the domination and control of everything in view. It is our particular social construction of reality that causes our estrangement, our homesickness, our civilizational emptiness. We create a reality divorced from nature, our life-world. We embrace instead the shopping mall with its myth of boundless economic growth and selfish fulfillment. It was all of this, the Bios say, that I began to sense in my early entries in this journal.

August 5th: The Bios continue to press the argument. In so doing, I see a whole worldview unfolding, a way of being in the world that we in the industrialized West have only rarely glimpsed. Yet it is a way of understanding the world that seems so right to me, so intuitively correct, that it is hard to ignore. Perhaps this is just what the Bios had in mind when they agreed to respect us as rational autonomous persons. Perhaps they know just how compelling their worldview can be, especially when seen against our own. But still the doubt lingers; are they manipulating?

Why then do these entries of the Bios' arguments seem as persuasive when I reread them? Is their manipulation that strong? After all, hasn't my own culture been manipulating my understanding all of my life? I'm a product of the very social construction of reality the Bios bemoan. Objectivity escapes us; that's what it means to be a person, a subject embedded in history. We only feign objectivity and, like the early arguments I gave about what is natural, confuse the objective point of view with the viewpoint that is dominant in our culture. As a result, we confuse the norm with the truth, the status quo with reality. It's a wonder we make any progress at all.

The Bios explained more fully how their notion of morality evolved from their notion of respect for nature.[10] The Bios acknowledge a hierarchy of actual interests within nature. Nonsentient life has an actual interest in the protection and pursuit of its own good, but it cannot be helped or harmed in terms of pleasure and pain. Hence, the moral consideration due to nonsentient life is more narrow than that due to sentient life. Sentient life has a greater capacity for help and harm, both qualitatively and quantitatively, because of its capacity for pleasure and pain.

Likewise, the moral consideration due to nonperson sentient beings is more narrow than that due to persons because the latter have the added capacity to be helped or harmed *vis-a-vis* their rational, valuing autonomy. Simply put, the hopes, dreams, and intentional aims of persons can be frustrated or aided in ways incompatible with creatures who lack the capacity for hopes, dreams, or intentional aims. Because our volitional life is richer, we have a greater capacity for help and harm than do creatures lacking our capacities. We must not forget that other life forms are due moral consideration; it is just not as broad as that due to persons. Although it is bad to take the life of any being, persons have fully fledged rights, including a fully fledged right to life.

Although we as persons, like all creatures, have a right of self-defense when our life is endangered, we are also constrained by a duty of noninterference in the life and ecosystems of other creatures when our life is not threatened. Although we have a right to protect and pursue our basic needs, those things necessary for us to live and flourish as rational, valuing beings who are autonomous centers of conscious life, we are constrained in our actions by the necessity to cause *minimum* damage to other life forms and the environment. Moreover, our right is to protect and pursue our *basic* needs. We have no right to protect and pursue nonbasic needs at the expense of other life forms or the environment. That is, we do not have the right to pursue either those particular ends that we desire or the means we consider best for achieving them, when those ends and means are not basic needs and when doing so is detrimental to other life or an ecosystem.

Hence, we as persons have a right to pursue food, fiber, and shelter, as well as love and personal relationships, as long as we do so in a manner that will minimize damage to the environment. Similarly we have a right to pursue whatever is necessary for us to

maintain and pursue our own good as a being; that is, our ration–
ality and autonomy. Doing so will obviously include the pursuit of
certain pleasures and satisfactions, as well as our own happiness, as
each of us as a valuing being define these. But in so doing, we are
constrained by the necessity to exact a minimum of damage on
nature in pursuit of our basic needs.[11]

So we should live, eat, and act to minimize harm to the actual
interests of other creatures while protecting and pursuing our own
good. It is this right, shared by all persons, that the Bios argue gives
them the right to use us, or at least some of us, for organ transplant.

Although it is always bad to use another creature as a mere
means, to fail to respect its own good, sometimes it is necessary in
order for another creature to continue its life. It is necessary for us
to take life for food in order to stay alive. This is justified on the
grounds of self-defense as long as we minimize harm to other life
and the environment, and make restitution for what we take.
Hence, vegetarianism is prescribed. Moreover, it should be a vege–
tarianism that minimizes harm to the environment and the needs of
other creatures, a vegetarianism based on small-scale, near self-
sufficient farming, the Bios argue.[12]

Similar to our need for food, the Bios find themselves in need of
organs if some of their members are to survive. As long as they
minimize the harm to other creatures and the environment, and
make restitution for what they take, they are, they claim, justified
in their actions. Unfortunately for us, humans are the only appropriate donors of which the Bios are aware.

All of this is, of course, more difficult because we are persons.
As such, we have a right to life over and above other moral claims.
Yet the Bios claim they want only those humans who are not
persons and who are unwanted by actual persons—unwanted
abortuses, babies, and mental defectives. Since these humans are
not persons, they do not have fully fledged rights nor a fully fledged
right to life. Since no actual person has an interest in them, no actual
person's autonomy will be violated by the Bios' actions. Moreover,
they claim that the proof of whether we care for or have an interest

in such a nonperson human is not merely our assent, but our willingness to provide for its basic needs, including its psychological needs for love and affection. Those who claim that fetuses and babies are the moral equal of a person need only provide the time and money necessary to care adequately for such nonperson humans in order to save them.

In return, the Bios will teach us how to perform abortions that are painless and harmless both to the mother and the unborn. They will remove from us the burden of providing, no matter how inadequately, for unwanted nonperson humans. They will continue to give us the ability, both intellectual and technological, although they assure us that we already have the latter, to adopt the attitudes of respect for nature, life, and persons.

Finally, they argue that although we may find their request morally grotesque, this is only because of our speciesism, our anthropocentrism, which is on a par with racism, sexism, classism, and nationalism. As evidence, they argue that we do not treat the baboons whose babies we steal to kill for organs with anything approaching the respect they offer to us. Let us not forget the whales and dolphins, the apes and chimps who we kill unnecessarily and whose environments we destroy needlessly. Then, of course, there are the countless animals we torture and kill through our attempts to dominate and subdue nature. Our speciesism re-veals itself at almost every turn in the moral argument and gives the lie to our claim of moral superiority to the Bios. Their biocentrism is, they claim, the broadest, most consistent, and most compelling moral perspective available.[13]

The history of persons throughout the universe reveals that the domain of the moral community is continually broadened as civilizations acquire greater understanding. The breadth of care seems to increase with the depth of knowledge. Human history is an excellent example. Over time, we have increased the moral community from members of our own clan, to city–states, to nation–states, and eventually, to the world of persons. Meanwhile, we have added people of differing religions, races, and gender to the moral community. We are beginning to take animals seriously as legitimate members of the moral community. Lately, arguments abound concerning the moral status of the unborn, the permanently comatose, and interplanetary aliens like the Bios. It should be apparent, the Bios argue, that our own moral evolution is quite simply retarded because of our speciesism and lack of respect for nature. It should come as no surprise, the Bios indicate, that our own moral future should be a biocentric one evidencing a deep care and respect for nature.

Postscript

Arguments, like the languages in which they have their life, only take on meaning within a context. I have tried to provide a different context, one that would force the reader to side not with those who desire to kill for the purpose of organ transplant, but instead with those who are to be killed. I want, quite simply, to encourage the reader to go beyond speciesism. Reversibility looms large in both the history and the logic of ethics. More importantly, it looms large in the moral and religious thought of almost all human cultures. I suspect that it is the *sine qua non* of the moral life.

What concerns me most with issues such as the use of animals for organ transplant is that to take such issues seriously is to see that a tragic flaw runs throughout Western moral theory. Why are we humans so special from a moral point of view? Is our insistence on our dominant moral standing anything more than an example of the Thrasymachan notion that justice is the interest of the stronger? Is it anything more than the denial of what we normally take to be the moral point of view? Is our insistence anything more than a reflection of the speciesism and resourcism generated by the melding of the medieval Judeo-Christian tradition with the rise of the new science during the Renaissance?[14] Why else would Eastern philosophies, which lack our tradition, tend to be so much less speciesist and resourcist? Does not this observation give the lie to the notion that Western moral theory is objective, ahistorical, and acultural? Does not this observation reveal instead that arguments, like the languages in which they have their life, take on meaning only within a context?

I have tried to present several different arguments and points of view concerning the morality of animal use for organ transplant. The initial position is one from the conservative right. It has its context within natural law theory and the notion of what is "natural." Of the three positions considered, the first is closest to common sense morality. Unfortunately, as indicated, the first position has all the weaknesses of any attempt to use the notions of the natural and the morally correct as one and the same. It is riddled with difficulties surrounding the meaning of "natural." Its persuasive definitions usually reduce to speciesism and an unjustified bias for the status quo.

The second position developed reflects a moderate or centrist position and is embedded within classical liberal notions of utilitarianism and rights. Although advanced by contemporary authors, these arguments reveal surprising similarities to the arguments of Bentham and Mill. They have many of the same faults.

To save the second position from collapse into the third, it is essential that one conflate having interests with forming perceived interests and persuasively define "good" and "bad" solely in terms of the experiences of sentient beings. Otherwise, there is no way to separate the moral standing of sentient life from nonsentient life. As I have indicated, I doubt that one can accomplish the conflation in any meaningful manner. I am strongly suspicious that the latter route leads to an unjustified bias for the sentient. Why should experience rather than life be central to morality? Surely we cannot reduce everything of value to experience.

As Taylor argues, all life seems to have inherent worth, to be due moral consideration solely for its own sake and in terms of its own good. Here the attitude of respect for life seems to be a rejection of the unjustified bias for the sentient for the same reason that other moral perspectives reject racism, sexism, classism, or speciesism.

The "ism" in question excludes others from moral standing for reasons that seem morally arbitrary.

The third argument yields conclusions compatible with the environmental left and with what is increasingly associated with the Green Party. It has the distinct disadvantage of contradicting common sense morality on some important issues like vegetarianism, the moral standing of nonsentient life, the moral standing of biotic communities, and the biosphere of the earth.[15] It is, however, remarkably consistent. A great deal of its counterintuitiveness concerning our treatment of nonperson humans and other animals is shared by the moderates.[16] But since such arguments aim at being revisionary rather than descriptive, these criticisms are external rather than internal ones. After all, a Green might argue, it is common sense morality that is largely responsible for the ecological and spiritual mess in which we presently find ourselves.[17]

I see the first conservative argument as a reflection of common sense morality, of conventional wisdom. Its failures give rise to the moderate liberal argument, the failings of which give rise to the third more radical view. Each argument negates the preceding one.

I draw no conclusions, although I clearly favor the arguments of the Bios. I do not see it as the job of the moral philosopher to draw moral conclusions, to tell other people what they ought to do, if for no other reason than they won't listen anyway. Moreover, it seems to me that they shouldn't listen when we tell them what to do. The important point is for one to develop one's own reflective morality, not to receive someone else's conventional wisdom. After all, we are rational, valuing beings who are autonomous centers of conscious life. We deserve to be treated as such, and one way to do so is to offer the reader a dialectic presentation of the issues for consideration.

Philosophy is an adept means of making evident the variety of possible positions and the numerous arguments that can be marshaled for and against the positions on many issues. Unfortunately, our clever manipulation of words and ideas cannot substitute for practical wisdom. When it is moral guidance that is needed, intelligence is no substitute for virtue. Consequently, we are usually confusing to the uninitiated. After all, they have not spent years in graduate school and the profession learning the proper universe of discourse, including its own rules for procedure and success. The uninitiated usually fail to understand what our language games have to do with morality. They understand that moral problems are not solved by thinking about them, that one does not become good merely by making the proper distinctions or learning a specialized set of language games. The uninitiated realize that moral problems are resolved through praxis. Most of all, they realize that moral judgment requires a good person rather than a clever or quick-witted one. What is needed is the manner and method of Socrates.

Notes and References

[1]Most parts of this entry are variations on themes by Peter Singer and Joel Feinberg. The latter is concerned primarily with issues of rights and interests, the former with the issues of speciesism, personhood, and sentiency. Peter Singer, *Animal Liberation.* New York: The New York Review, 1976 and "Not for Humans Only: The Place of Nonhumans in Environmental Issues," in K. C. Goodpaster and K. M. Sayre, eds., *Ethics and Problems of the 21st Century.* Notre Dame, Indiana: University of Notre Dame Press. Joel Feinberg, "The Rights of Animals and Unborn Generations." In William T. Blackstone, ed., *Philosophy and Environmental Crisis*, Athens, Georgia: The University of Georgia Press, 1974.

[2]It is not obvious that animals have the instinct to remain alive. They instinctively desire those things necessary to continue the species (e. g., food, drink, sex, natural habitat), which is a far different matter.

[3]Mary Ann Warren, "On the Moral and Legal Status of Abortion," *The Monist*, vol. 57, no. 1 (Jan. 1973), 43–61. It is also held by Peter Singer, *Practical Ethics.* Cambridge: Cambridge University Press, 1979. Similar views are held by Joel Feinberg, "Is There a Right to Be Born?" in *Understanding Moral Philosophy,* James Rachels, ed. Belmont, California: Dickenson Publishing, 1976. Notice that this view justifies abortion in cases where the mother has no interest in carrying the unborn to birth. It also justifies infanticide in those cases in which no person has an interest in caring for the infant.

[4]Joel Feinberg, 1974, for a discussion of the paradoxes of potentiality.

[5]The central arguments presented in the first half of this entry are, in the main, variations on themes found in Paul Taylor, *Respect for Nature,* Princeton: Princeton University Press, 1986.

[6]Taylor, p. 38. Although the notion of the attitude of respect for persons comes from Taylor, the argument advanced here to support it is actually a variation on Taylor's argument.

[7]The notion of respect for life is Taylor's. The argument for it diverges sharply from Taylor's more elaborate and detailed version, which is too involved to be condensed for this paper.

[8]The rest of this entry rests on variations on themes by Neil Evernden, *The Natural Alien,* Toronto: University of Toronto Press, 1985. This book reflects best my own view.

[9]Council on Environmental Quality and Department of State, *The Global 2000 Report to the President.* Robert L. Heilbroner, *An Inquiry Into the Human Prospect,* NY: W. W. Norton, 1975.

[10]The arguments of this section return to variations on themes by Taylor.

[11]The clash of duties that results from the conflicting claims of different species is handled at greater length and depth by Taylor than I can cover here. See particularly chapter 6, but also 4 and 5. There he develops a hierarchy of moral principles to adjudicate moral disputes across species.

[12]See Francis Moore Lappe (1975)*Diet for a Small Planet,* New York. rev. ed; Francis Moore Lappe and Joseph Collins, *Food First,* Boston: Houghton Mifflin, 1975.

[13]See Taylor's arguments for the respect for nature and Singer on speciesism for elaboration on the points made here.

[14]I take resourcism to be the view that nature is a lifeless, boundless storehouse to be dominated and controlled, that is, exploited, to serve human interests.

[15]Although beyond the scope of this paper, the worldview of the Bios is, I believe, consistent with moderate views on abortion based on the developing sentiency of the unborn. See my, "The Ontological and Moral Standing of the Unborn," *Today's Moral Problems,* 2nd ed, Richard Wasserstrom, ed. New York: Macmillan Publishing, 1979; or L. W. Sumner, *Abortion and Moral Theory,* Princeton: Princeton University Press, 1981.

[16]See previous points on Singer and Feinberg, particularly note 3.

[17]Rudolh Bahro, *Socialism and Survival.* London: Heretic Books, 1982; Carl Boggs, "The Greens," *Our Generation,* vol. 18, no. 1 (Fall/Winter 1986), pp. 1–61.

Animal Parts, Human Wholes

*On the Use of Animals as a Source
of Organs for Human Transplants*

R. G. Frey

Is the use of animals as a source of organs for human transplants morally permissible? I think that such use is or can be permissible; but, as with my defense of vivisection in "Vivisection, Medicine, and Morals," in the *Journal of Medical Ethics*,[1] and in my book, *Rights, Killing, and Suffering*,[2] I also think that this permissibility can only be obtained at a cost that few people appear prepared to pay. I am not prepared to pay it indiscriminately, without regard to the nature and extent of the benefit to be derived in the particular case; and I do not think one *can* pay this price in the animal case without being prepared to pay it in the cases of some humans. In a word, I do not think we can use animals as a resource for humans without being prepared to use some humans as a resource for humans; and if the benefit to be derived in the particular case can make the use of animals appear worth it, so the benefit can make the use of humans appear worth it.

I do not wish to discuss the issue of benefit here, and, indeed, in an important sense, it is not of fundamental concern. For in order to raise the question of whether it is morally permissible to use animals as a resource for humans, we may make almost any assumption we like about benefit, given that, without some prospect of benefit to the human, the transplant would not have been undertaken or contemplated in the first place. Discussion of the case of Baby Fae has been preoccupied with a host of doubts about the appropriateness of xenograft, medically, and about the prospective benefit to the infant that xenograft was likely to confer. (As is well-known, of course, the case gave rise to other issues, such as the presence or absence of informed consent, the extent of the search for a child donor, and the possible, antecedent commitment of Dr. Leonard Bailey and his team to xenograft.) Certainly, from all that I have read, the transplantation of a baboon heart into Baby Fae, particularly in the light of the history of negative results of xenograft, justifiably raised questions of appropriateness. Yet, the fact that Baby Fae lived only two weeks or so with her new heart, the supposed benefit, is in an important sense not of fundamental concern here; for even if she had lived for a much longer time or, indeed, had survived for a very considerable period, we should still be entitled to ask whether this use of an animal for human purposes was justifiable. Dr. Jack W. Provonsha suggests that, because Baby Fae had "at least two good weeks" after surgery and lived longer "than any other xenograft had ever survived," she gained from the transplant.[3] I am far from clear that "two good weeks" counts as much of a benefit in the case of a 15-day-old girl, and I am very far from clear that "two good weeks" in the case of a 15-day-old girl makes it worth depriving an otherwise healthy baboon of its life. The unthinking assumption, that the extension of any human life for any period of time whatever is a benefit, is not one I share; accordingly, I do not share the view that a series of operations on a severely handicapped newborn in order to prolong its life by a few months is obviously a benefit to the infant.

As I say, however, the question of benefit can be left aside here. For what motivates our concern now is not really the success or failure of our using animals as a resource, but rather the moral permissibility of our making use of them in the first place. Thus, cardiac surgeons transplant pig valves into humans with success, with consequent prolongation of life; but success does not mean that we do not have to face the question of whether it is morally permissible for us to use pigs in this way. Plainly, success may make it easier for us to convince ourselves that our use of animals *is* permissible, a possibility to which we must remain alert; but it cannot dissolve the issue of use or remove from us the necessity of dealing with it.

I have said that benefit is not the fundamental notion upon which the subject of our use of animals turns. In my view, the morality of using animals as a resource for human transplants and the morality of xenograft itself, as with the morality of vivisection, turn fundamentally upon the comparative worth of animal and human life. I do not claim that other issues to do with these practices may be ignored; but I do indeed think that until we decide the comparative value of animal and human life, the morality of these practices will never be finally resolved. What they are centrally about, as I have indicated, is the deliberate and extensive use of one or more species by another, and the only thing that can justify this sort of usage, I think, is a difference in value between animal and human life.

I have tried in the material cited above, especially in *Rights, Killing, and Suffering*, to argue for a marked difference between the value of animal and normal human life, and, importantly, in a way that avoids the charge of speciesism. More recently, I have deepened and extended my account of the matter in forthcoming papers on "Autonomy and The Value of Animal Life,"[4] "The Significance of Agency and Marginal Cases,"[5] and "Autonomy and Conceptions of the Good Life."[6] All this fresh material sets still further apart the value of animal and normal human life, by (i) contrasting the quality and richness of animal and human life over a wide spectrum, (ii) setting out how autonomy typically enables humans to add new dimensions of value to their lives, and (iii) showing that animals are not autonomous in any sense that does justice to our understanding of why autonomy is an immensely important value.[7] I do not have space here to repeat the arguments of either the earlier or this fresh material; but I do not need to, I think, in order to be able to show how the very inegalitarianism between the value of animal and human life that justifies our making use of animals equally justifies our making use of some humans.

I stress that my concern here is with the question of our using animals; I have nothing to say, therefore, on the horror that some people purport to experience at the mere thought of cross-transplantion, of grafting animal organs into humans. Again, my concern is with the extreme case of using animals for human transplants, in which, as with the case of Baby Fae, an animal is killed in order to try to save a human. For I take killing members of another species in order to try to save members of our own to be the ultimate usage our species can make of another; and I assume that, if this ultimate usage of a species can be justified, then some less ultimate usage of it can be justified. Finally, it is important to be sensitive to the possibility that many people who oppose killing animals for food or in tests of cosmetics or detergents or in much medical experimentation or for furs may well have a different view of the use of animals to save human lives. In this event, it becomes important to go into just how likely it is that the use of animal organs will save the human life in question; that is, into just how realizable and substantial a benefit the transplant may be expected to produce. And a host of other issues arise as well. The point is that many people may well regard the killing of animals to save human lives in a quite different light from other uses we make of animals; but such people too, I believe, will rest their case in whole or in part upon the difference in value between animal and human life.

Killing and the value of life are connected, since if a particular life had no value it is difficult to see why taking it would be wrong. Very few people, I suspect, think animal life to be of no value, so that we need not bother ourselves about taking it; but equally few people, I believe, think that animal life has the same value as normal human life. On the value of these lives, we are not egalitarians. Nor do we run afoul of the charge of speciesism thereby: for reasons I have set out in the material cited above, we regard normal human life to be of a much higher quality than animal life, not because of species, but because of richness; and the value of life is a function of its quality. As a result, and this is the important point, the threshold for killing animals is lower than that for killing normal adult humans.

To be sure, part of the richness of our lives involves activities we have in common with animals; but the truth is that we engage in a whole host of activities—falling in love, marrying, helping our children and young people to grow in numerous ways, working well and achieving job satisfaction, developing our minds in ways our relations never thought possible, acquiring cultural and intellectual interests, as well as hobbies, that expand our range of absorbing experiences in life, and so on—that immeasurably deepen the texture of our lives. (I discuss this matter in some detail in the material already cited.) The lives of normal adult humans betray a richness and variety that the lives of (infants, defective humans, and) animals do not; thus, we are not condemned, in the sense intended, to live out our lives according to our species or to seek no further than the lives of our ancestors or those around us for models by which to live. As I have remarked in several places, when we say of a person that he or she has led a rich, full life, we refer to something incomparably beyond what we would refer to were we to say the same of a chicken or cat.

The point is not that the activities that enrich a human's life *are different from* those that enrich a chicken's life; it is that the scope or potentiality for enrichment is truncated or severely diminished in the chicken's case. In my view, the value of life is a function of its quality, its quality a function of its richness, and its richness a function of its scope or potentiality for enrichment; and the scope or potentiality for enrichment in the chicken's case never approaches that of the human. This can be seen quite readily if we look at the role autonomy plays in our lives.

Autonomy—whether construed as personhood and acting as a person, self-determination, choice, or adopting and living out a life plan, all of which rely upon or involve agency—is a value to which moral theorists of all stripes today give great prominence, and, at least in the context of my own views, it is easy to understand why. By exercising our autonomy, we can mould our lives to fit a conception of the good life that we have decided upon for ourselves; we can then seek to live out this conception, with the strong sense of achievement, self-fulfillment, and satisfaction that this can bring. We can work long and hard at some athletic, cultural, or intellectual endeavour and take satisfaction in the self-fulfillment and sense of accomplishment that (relative) success brings. The emphasis is upon agency: we can *mold* or *shape* our lives into the lives of athletes, musicians, or educators; by exercising our autonomy, that is, we can *impose upon our lives* a conception of the good life and then seek to live out that conception, with the consequent sense of self-fulfillment and achievement that this makes possible. These things in turn typically are sources of immense satisfaction to us. Thus, by exercising our autonomy and trying to live out a conception of the good life, we make possible a further and important dimension of value to our lives. And most of us do this; for adopting and living out some conception of the good life need not be something that requires deep thought. Yet, it does require thought, and we do have to work at the matter; for we do have to mold or shape our lives to "fit" our conception of the good life. To live out a conception of the good life involves turning one's life into a life appropriate to the conception involved. A professional musician has to turn his life into that of a professional musician; the life of a professional athlete would not enable him to live the life most conducive to being a professional musician.

To the above, nothing comparable exists among animals and other non-autonomous creatures[8]; and this fact provides an additional reason for thinking their lives are less rich than the lives of normal adult humans. In the case of autonomy, what is missing is the same scope or potentiality for enrichment; and lives of less richness have less value. Therefore, since the rightness of killing is related to the value of the life taken, since autonomy matters to the value of life, and since the lives of the nonautonomous are less valuable than the lives of the autonomous, the threshold for taking the lives of non-autonomous beings is lower than that for taking the lives of autonomous ones. Here again, then, we reach the conclusion that the threshold for killing animals is lower than that for killing normal adult humans.

It is important to guard against two mistakes that are frequently made at this point. First, there has been a wholesale effort of late to show that, although animals are not moral agents, nevertheless they are members of the moral community. Such membership alone, however, does not answer to present purposes: even if animals *are* members of the moral community, it does not follow that their lives are of equal value to the lives of normal adult humans. *Are* animals members of the moral community? Let us concede that they are; after all, they can suffer and suffering is an evil. Nevertheless, it does not follow from the fact that they can suffer that animals have lives of (roughly) equal value to those of normal adult humans.

Importantly, this result fits nicely with the discussion of autonomy. I do not think animals are autonomous in any sense that even remotely captures our understanding of why autonomy is such an immensely important value; but I also do not think the possession of autonomy is a *sine qua non* condition for admission to the moral community. The sufferings of non-autonomous beings count morally, but, to repeat, it still does not follow that they have lives of (roughly) equal value to those of normal adult humans. Autonomy is related to the value of life, not to membership in the moral community.

The second mistake is to assume that the lives of all *human* members of the moral community are of equal value. It is my rejection of this assumption that leads directly to the corollary of my conclusion in the case of animals: the threshold for taking the lives of severely defective humans is lower than that for taking the lives of normal adult humans. The truth is that it is not only animals who have lives of less value than normal adult humans; so, too, do some humans. This fact in turn destroys the basis for any argument from marginal cases, since if not all human life has the same value, the cases of deficient human life cannot be used to force the concession of equal value for the lives of animals.

Any number of humans lead lives of considerably lower quality than ordinary human lives, lives that not only lack much richness, but also lack the scope or potentialities for enrichment of normal lives. The temptation always is to go to cases of the irreversibly comatose for examples; but we need not. The very severely mentally enfeebled, the seriously brain damaged, severely handicapped newborns, such as those born with no or only half a brain or with hypoplastic left heart syndrome, elderly people fully in the grip of Alzheimer's disease, people dying in the final stages of cardiomyopathy—all kinds of examples, and in almost limitless numbers, come to mind. If the value of a life is a function of its quality, and if there are humans whose lives are of a very much lower quality than ordinary human life, then some human lives have less value than others. Depending upon how severely impaired those lives are, they can fall so far below the quality of ordinary human life as to become lives that we would not wish ourselves to live and that we would not wish to compel anyone else to live and so to become lives that we may come to think are not worth living. (It remains a mystery to me, therefore, as to why some people seem driven to compel severely handicapped newborns to undergo one operation after another, in the hope of conferring upon these infants some further, usually short, period of massively impoverished life.) In particular, the quality of a human life can fall to a point that the life of a healthy baboon can seem readily to equal, or, indeed, exceed it, can seem not worth sacrificing in order to save the human life. Only, then, if one invokes the dictum that a human life of any quality, however low, exceeds in value an animal life of any quality, however high, can one ensure that human life will always remain more valuable; but I myself can see no reason whatever to accept any such dictum. It seems to me to represent a form of speciesism, at least on any obvious understanding of it.

In no way does the above commit one to the view that, e.g., the very severely mentally enfeebled, elderly people fully in the grip of Alzheimer's disease and severely handicapped newborns are not members of the moral community; all, I presume, can suffer. (I have not space to consider the cases of beings that cannot suffer.) The above does commit one to the view, however, that not all human life has the same value. If, then, we retain the view that the morality of killing is linked to the value of the life taken, we seem forced to conclude that the threshold for killing severely defective humans is lower than that for killing normal adult humans.[9]

It is easy now to see the rationale behind my position on vivisection. Experimentation on animals for human benefit is nearly always justified by appeal to the difference in value between their lives; but the lives of some humans are of a quality comparable to or even below that of many of the healthy animals on whom the experiments are performed. Why, then, not perform the experiments on the humans? The benefit to be derived could be equally, if not better, obtained, since often the extrapolation of results from animal to human cases is not very reliable. In *Rights, Killing, and Suffering*, I envisage some of the appeals to side effects that might be made to bar the human experiments; after all, it seems likely that many people would be outraged by such experiments and would be reluctant to go into hospital and to be attended by medical people.[10] Side effects, however, may or may not arise; certainly, they seem at least in many cases to be susceptible to removal by education, information, and careful explanation of the arguments.

I should stress that I do not welcome human experiments; I endorse them very reluctantly. But if we are going to continue to perform experiments on healthy animals and attempt to justify them by appeal to the value of their lives, then I can see no way consistently to avoid experiments upon humans. For I cannot think of anything at all compelling that cedes human life of any quality greater value than animal life of any quality. Clearly, we have here a powerful argument for antivivisectionism: it is one sure way to bar human experiments. The reason I cannot endorse it is that it looks in the face the benefits to be derived from (some, by no means all) experimentation.[11] (I do not here take a stand on how far the search for replacements of animals in research has progressed, for us to conclude that the extent and variety of information to be derived from those replacements enables us to forego further animal experimentation. Certainly, I welcome the search for replacements.)

What is true of animal experimentation is true of the use of animals as a source of organs for human transplants: virtually every defence of this practice I have seen appeals directly or indirectly to the value of animal life. As a result, I can see no way consistently to bar using some humans in this way, since, to repeat, I can think of nothing at all compelling that cedes human life of any quality greater value than animal life of any quality. Indeed, I can think of a powerful reason favoring the use of humans. The history of xenograft is not one of marked success, and cross-species transplantation of vital organs at the moment seems far less likely to produce benefit than transplantation from one human to another. Thus, if one *were* going to make the discussion turn upon realizable benefit, then the use of humans as a source of organs seems demanded.

Of course, it may be objected that we already experiment upon some humans and use some humans as organ donors for others; but I take it that there is a clear difference between the animal and human case in this regard. Consent is required from the human or his or her trustee; the animal is seized and used. It will be urged that the animal cannot consent; but how does lack of consent, then, justify going ahead and using the animal? The very severely mentally enfeebled cannot consent, yet that fact is not at present taken as a justification for using their organs. Again, it might be urged that the crucial difference is that the trustee or family of the severely mentally enfeebled person would not consent. I think we can see that consent is not the vital issue in all this, however, by simply supposing that the trustee or family did give their consent to use the person as a source of organs: I think a great many people would still insist that it would be wrong to use a human being in this way. What underlies their view either directly or indirectly, I believe, is their conviction that human life is more valuable than animal life and so cannot be used in ways that animal life can; it is this conviction that I reject, not by denying that much human life is more valuable than animal life, but by denying that all is. Certainly, we owe severely deficient humans charity; but, again, I can see no good reason to think that we do not owe animals charity.

In my view, then, we cannot use animals as a resource for humans without being prepared to use some humans as a resource for humans. The humans to be used are those with a very low quality of life, in which the scope or potentiality for enrichment is severely truncated or absent, as in the cases presented above. Any life about which there is much doubt in this regard is not to be regarded as a resource. Let me now link this view to the specifics of the situation surrounding xenograft.

What fuels the drive to reliance upon xenograft is the abundance of potential animal organs. This is another way of alluding to shortages of human organs, to, in other words, the relative scarcity of human donors. The fewer the number of human donors of organs for transplant, the greater the attraction use of animals presents. One can attack this problem of shortages by using animal organs or by trying to increase the number of human donors (or, of course, by employing both means). All the evidence to date suggests better results attend the use of human donors, not xenograft; so the campaign to increase the number of human donors—to urge people to save or improve lives through donating their or their family members' organs upon death—needs our best efforts.

The argument of this paper suggests at once three directions in which this campaign should move.

Harvesting the Biological Dead

Here, for humans, quality of life considerations have been extinguished, and the scope or potentiality for enrichment of life has gone entirely. A life has ceased to have value, and this seems to imply two things. First, the organs of the biological dead become obvious resources for human transplants, in a context in which the removal and use of those organs can in no way diminish the quality, and so the value, of the lives of the biological dead. Second, and much more importantly, this first point means that it would be wrong to use the organs of healthy animals *instead of* or *in order to avoid the use of* the organs of the biological dead. Unlike the case of the biological dead, the removal of organs from an otherwise healthy animal does indeed diminish the quality and value of its life, and there seems no justification for this, at least if we take the appeal to the value of life seriously.

The central problem with harvesting the organs of dead people is, obviously, not with the dead person, but with the living; *their* quality of life, they may urge, is adversely affected by treating their relation as a resource. It is here that the education campaign must be especially forthcoming.

The campaign must not only urge people to become organ donors upon death, but also instill in them the importance of coming to adopt a view of the dead person as a main source of life, and improvement of life, for others. To be asked for the organs of a loved one immediately upon their death can be a very upsetting experience; to be of use, the organs must be removed more or less at once, and family members may not have had time to take in, let alone accept, their loss. Again, for all the complexity of the many contemporary discussions of personhood and personal identity, many people still identify the person with the body. As a result, cutting open the body can be seen as a direct assault upon the person one has loved, and it is not easy to bring oneself to accept, as it were, the partial, physical destruction of that in which one has invested one's deepest affections. Much more of a similar kind could be said; all of it indicates how difficult it will be to change people's perception of the dead body. Yet, the tragedy that death brings a family need not mean a tragedy for another family as well, if the dead body can come to be regularly perceived as a source of life or of the enhancement of life for others.

Finally, it should be noted that, however difficult it may be to bring about a change in our perception of the dead body, harvesting the organs of the biological dead does not involve killing anyone. This is a marked difference between using animals and using the biological dead as resources, and it should be possible with an education campaign to build upon this difference, in favor of the use of the biological dead.

Harvesting the Brain Dead

What is true in the case of the biological dead is true in the case of the brain dead: quality of life considerations are no longer applicable, and the scope or potentiality for enriching the life in question has disappeared. Here, too, then, humans become obvious resources for human transplants, in a context in which the removal and use of their organs does not diminish the quality and value of the lives in question. Thus, once again, it would be wrong to use the organs of healthy animals *instead of* or *in order to avoid the use of* the organs of the brain dead. The removal of organs from an otherwise healthy animal does indeed diminish the quality and value of its life, something that the appeal to quality of life seems unable to justify, in the presence of the brain dead.

Some might insist that, because the brain dead are not biologically dead, it is not strictly true that quality of life considerations cannot apply in their cases. This line of argument does not alter the situation *vis-à-vis* animals, however, since it seems very clear that the quality of life of a healthy primate or animal generally is considerably higher than that of the brain dead. In which case, the appeal to the value of life would still favor harvesting the organs of the brain dead.

A great deal has been written about brain death and its replacement of biological death as our criterion for what it is to die. An education campaign will certainly have fully to explore the issues involved and seek to bring people to realize the positions of the brain dead and animals with respect to harvesting organs for transplant. I suspect the hardest part of the campaign will be to change the perception of the brain dead as in something akin to a deep sleep. On the sleep model, one can hope that the brain dead will awaken, whereas, of course, one cannot hold out any such hope in the case of the biological dead. This hope is an important part of us, something we cherish; it is akin to our hope in certain medical cases that some discovery will tonight be made that saves our relation. The problem with the sleep model is that it lends itself to a failure on our parts to realize what brain death typically means in a case. Severe brain damage, deterioration of the nervous system, degeneration of organs, atrophy of neural and other functions— what would come out of the deep sleep would be a very severely impoverished version of what went into it. Thus, of ordinary sleep, one can easily understand the claim that the functions and potentialities of the enrichment of a life remain present in the sleeping person, to become manifest when the person awakes. In the deep sleep of the brain dead, however, in which deterioration and atrophy of organs and functions is typically the case, it is far from clear what such a claim could mean. And the longer the period of brain death, the even more remote it becomes that such a claim could be true.

Harvesting the Living

Here we come to the cases discussed earlier in this paper, to people who are not biologically dead or brain dead, but whose lives are of a very low quality and in which the scope or potentiality for enrichment is severely truncated or absent. Since I have already discussed these cases, I shall only remark here that the position with respect to animals seems clear. If we are going to justify the use of animals as resources for human transplants by appeal to the value of their lives, then we seem committed to the justification of the use of those humans whose lives are roughly commensurate in value to or fall below the value of the lives of animals. The only way I can see to avoid this commitment is to cite something that makes it the case that a human life of any quality, even if disastrously low, has greater value than an animal life of any quality, even if extraordinarily high. I can think of nothing at all compelling to cite in this regard. By parity of reasoning with the biological and brain dead cases, therefore, it would be wrong to use the organs of healthy animals *instead of* or *in order to avoid the use of* the organs of severely deficient humans whose lives are of a very low quality and where the scope or potentiality for enrichment is severely truncated or absent.

Thus, the use of severely deficient humans, harvesting them for their organs, must be envisaged and implemented, if (i) one tries to justify such a use of animals on the basis of the value of their lives, (ii) one cannot say anything at all compelling to show that human life of any quality has greater value than animal life of any quality, and (iii) one proceeds with the use of animals. Obviously, one does not welcome the use of humans as a human resource, but neither, I hope, does one *welcome* the use of animals as a human resource. Moreover, the claim that it is *necessary* to use animals as a source of organs is clearly false. It is only necessary to use them *if* one does not use humans.

In the case of Baby Fae, then, imagine the following situation: in one room is a perfectly healthy baboon, in another is a very severely handicapped infant, say, one born without a brain. If Dr. Bailey is to proceed with the transplant at all, he can kill the baboon and use its heart or kill the infant and use its heart (which is unaffected by the infant's brain condition). If one truly is going to appeal to the value of life to decide the case, then I cannot see that killing the baboon is justified, especially if the education campaign to help dissipate the side-effects of using the infant has been undertaken seriously. I recognize that this conclusion will be very unpalatable to many, but I can, in the context I have discussed, see no way of avoiding it.

Of course, it may well be said that what is needed is a heavy dose of fellow-feeling; the problem is to understand how fellow-feeling enters the argument.

In one obvious form, the claim comes unstuck. If by "fellow-feeling" is meant positive feelings of good will toward others, then one must contend with the fact, or so it appears to me, that few seem to betray such feelings *to the world at large*, let alone to betray them when their own interests are threatened. The father who donates a kidney to save his daughter does not do so to save a stranger—or a more remote relative. If, however, by "fellow-feeling" is meant merely being affected in some degree by what befalls others, then one must contend with the facts (i) that we are affected by the plight of animals, particularly the higher ones, and (ii) that merely being affected by the plight of others often does not of itself motivate us to do anything about their condition, does not of itself, in other words, indicate anything positive at all about some natural propensity of ours to assist our fellow humans. We are all aware of the plight of the starving poor, in this age of television; the fact remains that, although affected, few of us contribute, and very few of us contribute substantially, to relieve their condition. Thus, it is hard to see how the fact that we are affected by the plight of others can be taken to show anything at all about some natural propensity of ours to prefer the well-being of others or even to prefer that these others live.

It is tempting to take the charge about fellow-feeling to be a demand directly to inject a factor of bias in favor of our own kind into the argument. Exactly how one injects such a factor is a very important matter, a consideration of which must await another occasion; here, I want only to point to the obvious fact that a good deal turns upon how one interprets the expression "our own kind." As I have said, I take seriously the charge of speciesism; I think discrimination solely on the basis of species is wrong. The trick for one who would inject such a bias into the argument is to do so in a way that avoids the charge of speciesism, and the problem that then ensues is to inject a bias in favor of species in a way that does not permit biases in favor of race, gender, or religion also to be injected into the argument. All of these represent possible interpretations of the phrase "our own kind," and it is far from clear how one interpretation can be admissible but all others barred.

There is a further difficulty here that those who would inject a bias in favor of species into the argument must address. Virtually every such attempt with which I am familiar tries to move from cases involving special relationships—the father donates his kidney to save his daughter, but not a stranger—to some general claim about favoring our species. That is, if the father can favor his child and have this count as moral, why cannot we favor members of our own species and have that count as moral? At least part of the reason has to do with the very item mentioned: although the parent stands in a special relationship to the child, we all do not stand in a special relationship to each other. The way the favor shown the child comes to be moral is by means of the special relation in which the parent stands to the child; typically, we do not stand to each other in any special relationship whatever. Mere membership in the moral community does not form a special relationship; but even if it did, since animals are members of the moral community, we acquire no ground for differentiating human from animal cases. Thus, it seems to me that what one is forced into defending is the claim that being members of the same species constitutes a special relationship. I do not have space to discuss this matter here, but I doubt the truth of this claim and for a variety of reasons. For example, a special relationship with someone is typically, as it were, something we step into and, in time, can step out of; but species membership is not something we step into or out of at all, not something we voluntarily acquire in any way whatever, and so not something we think of in moral terms at all. Again, to have a special relationship that is outside our control—we do not choose our species membership— is an unusual conception of such a relationship as it is of moral relations generally. Much more could be said. The point is that argument is needed to show that mere species membership is a special, moral relationship in which all humans stand to each other. One must be careful not to confuse this view with the claim that all persons, to the extent that they are able, have a duty to render mutual aid to each other. I know of no defense of this latter claim that grounds such a duty in *species* membership. It may turn out that only humans are persons and that, therefore, only humans have duties of mutual aid; but the ground of that duty or the reason humans have it is not the fact that or because they are members of the same species *homo sapiens*.

One final point. I do not accept the view that the extension of any human life for any period of time whatever is a benefit; the reader will have gathered why from the arguments of this paper. Yet, I think this view is widespread among medical and nonmedical people alike, and acceptance of it creates pressure for more and more transplants, whether of hearts, kidneys, livers, and so on. Our education campaign must not only examine very thoroughly the benefit to be gained by transplant, the resources to be expended in gaining that benefit, and the question of whether that benefit is worth that cost; it must also, in order to decide this last question, examine the assumption that the prolongation of life is *per se* a benefit. To prolong life regardless of quality is not *per se* to confer a benefit, and on this ground alone transplant cases need to be closely examined.

Notes and References

[1]"Vivisection, Medicine, and Morals" *in Journal of Medical Ethics*, vol. 9, 1983, pp. 94–104. Reprinted in *Bioethics Reporter*, no. 2, 1984.

[2]*Rights, Killing, and Suffering* (Oxford, Basil Blackwell, 1983), especially ch. 12 ("The Value of Life").

[3]Jack W. Provonsha, "Was It Ethical To Implant A Baboon Heart In Baby Fae?," in Carol Levine (ed.), *Taking Sides: Clashing Views On Controversial Bioethical Issues*, 2nd ed. (Gailford, CN, Dushkin Publishing Group, 1987), p. 222.

[4]"Autonomy and The Value of Animal Life," in *The Monist*, forthcoming (special issue on animal rights).

[5]"The Significance of Agency and Marginal Cases," in *Philosophica*, forthcoming (special issue on environmental ethics).

[6]"Autonomy and Conceptions of The Good Life," in T. Attig, and D.Callan, L.W. Sumner (eds.), *Values and Moral Standing*, Bowling Green Applied Philosophy Program, forthcoming.

[7]In "Autonomy and The Value of Animal Life," *op. cit.*, I try to show why Tom Regan's view (*The Case for Animal Rights*, Berkeley, University of California Press, 1983) of autonomy in animals will not do.

[8]I discuss this matter more thoroughly in my papers "Autonomy and The Value of Animal Life" and "The Significance of Agency and Marginal Cases," *op. cit.*

[9]I attack Regan's claims about the value and the equal inherent value of human life in "Autonomy and The Value of Animal Life," *op. cit.*

[10]See *Rights, Killing, and Suffering, op. cit.*, ch. 12.

[11]I am indebted in this discussion of harvesting the dead to work by Joel Feinberg and to a conference paper by Robert Hallborg, Jr., presented in Bowling Green in 1986.

Animals as a Source of Human Transplant Organs

James L. Nelson

Introduction

The transplantation of whole organs—liver, kidneys, and even hearts—has quickly become a familiar part of medicine's repertoire. But it is nonetheless hampered by a number of serious problems. Some are technical; of these, the most prominent concerns the management of the body's tendency to reject tissues it considers foreign. Problems of this sort are better understood than once they were; the recent development of cyclosporine A, a powerful immunosuppressant drug, has had in particular a great influence on the growth of organ transplantion to a mature therapy.[1]

Other problems occasioned by organ transplantation are ethical; they include such things as standards of informed consent for donors and recipients, and criteria for the just allocation of scarce resources. Perhaps the most crucial problem of this kind is that of obtaining donors in sufficient number to meet a demand whose growth seems assured.

And there is also, of course, a meta-problem: should we remain wedded to the current approach to health care, stressing technology-intensive cures rather than prevention, which involves a markedly anti-egalitarian distribution of resources, or should we shift our allegiance to a more socially oriented conception of good health, underscoring health education and prophylaxis? The future of organ transplantation is clearly bound up with our continuing in something closely resembling the present medical style.

Problems such as these tend to resist definitive solutions; there is no ethical cyclosporine A on the horizon. So it would seem altogether reasonable to sidestep whatever ethical problems one can, and to transfer the burden to the technical end. The use of animals as a source of human transplant organs can be seen as a response to the problem of obtaining suitable organs in sufficient numbers. Procurement is a serious problem, and only in part because the process of obtaining human organs is in general an inefficient one. The situation is clearly summarized in a recent article by Arthur Caplan, who notes that "even if the current system of procuring organs from cadaver sources were modified so as to increase the efficiency of cadaver organ procurement, there would still exist a significant shortfall in the number of kidneys, livers, and hearts available for transplantation to children and adults."[2] The appeal of xenograft is that it reduces the procurement problem by a considerable amount, although the primate of choice in human-animal xenograft, the chimpanzee, is extremely difficult to obtain.[3] It also makes the availability of organs a more stable matter; nonhuman animals, unlike their human counterparts, can be held at the ready for the express purpose of organ donations.

It is some measure of how attractive these considerations are that we are willing to shoulder the technical burdens involved. They become more onerous the further genetically the recipient is from the donor. "Autograft"—the transplantation of organs or tissues from one site on the body to another—is in general the simplest procedure, since there is no danger of the body rejecting its own tissue. This is also the case when the donor is the recipient's identical twin. "Allograft," or transplantation between genetically distinct individuals, is much trickier, since the possibility of rejection is quite real, and tends to become more likely the greater the difference between the parties to the transaction. This is the ground on which interfamilial transplants have been preferred.[4]

The limit case of allograft is xenograft, the transplantation of organs or tissues from a member of one species to a member of another. At the level of whole organs and with human subjects, it is a technique much more discussed than practiced; when it has been employed, the results have been uniformly unsatisfactory. The case of Baby Fae is well known; Fae's transplant was preceded in the 1960s by much more obscure, but equally unsuccessful, essays in cardiac and renal xenotransplantation.[5] Tissue and bone xenografts are more common—sheep intestine is used for surgical sutures, tendons and bones from cows have replaced human ones, and valves from the hearts of pigs have been used to repair human hearts.[6] These successful efforts in the art of inter-species transplantation suggest that major organ xenograft might evolve from its present almost desperately unsatisfactory, highly experimental state, to a therapeutic resource that could be applied with some confidence, especially in cases like Baby Fae's.

Fae was born with a congenital heart defect called hypoplastic left heart syndrome, or HLHS.[7] This defect is invariably fatal; conventional surgical techniques are of little value. Children in Fae's position are candidates for heart transplant, but as Senator Albert Gore pointed out in a recent Hastings Center Report discussion of Fae's case, trauma deaths in infants are (thankfully) rare, and children in Fae's condition cannot wait.[8] If animals could be used as a source of organs for humans, the supply problem would become much more tractable, more a matter of economics than anything else. And this happy result might be extendable to diseases other than HLHS, mitigating serious ethical problems of allocation and consent.

Xenograft is not without its own moral problems, of course. Some have arisen in particular instances; in the Baby Fae case, for example, the NIH team visiting Loma Linda Medical Center were critical of what they saw as overstatement of the likely benefits from xenograft, and general questions have been raised about the vigor with which a human cadaver heart was sought. Other concerns range more generally over xenograft. They include:

Microallocation questions. Insofar as all or some xenografts (particularly in the developmental stage of this therapy) are seen as stopgap implants, maintaining an individual until human organs are available, similar questions to those asked in artificial heart usage arise. Such temporary use of animal or artificial organs puts patients in a state of medical emergency, and may unjustly skew the distribution of human organs in their favor.

Economic questions. If, either presently or in the future, xenografts are offered without cost, or at a reduced cost, compared to allografts, while at the same time constituting a less satisfactory therapy, questions about both the validity of informed consent and justice in the distribution of medical resources arise.[9]

Moral psychological questions. It is worth wondering what impact the availability of animal organs may have on the altruistic dispositions that incline people to make anatomical gifts. In the light of the perception that human donations were not strictly necessary, might such donations fall off more precipitously than the existing xenographic resources could accommodate? Might the ultimate success of xenograft take from us an important opportunity to express altruism, to make to those who are strangers, but yet members of the moral community, a gift of great significance, to invest our deaths with meaning?

But the most serious of the moral complexities with which xenograft is entangled may not be located in considerations of consent, or of justice in allocation, or in its impact on our moral sensibilities. Rather, the most serious source of moral problems here may come from a buried premise in the notion that xenograft is, at least ultimately, morally less costly than human allograft, viz., that animals are not morally considerable beings. For if they are to be taken seriously from a moral viewpoint, the entire proposal needs to be reexamined—as does medical and scientific research overall.[10]

The past decade or so has seen an unprecedented amount of interest in the question of what is morally owing to animals. The next section of this essay surveys some of the most important results to emerge from these investigations.

The Moral Standing of Animals

In a recent working paper, Tom L. Beauchamp notes the progress in our understanding of the moral constraints surrounding experimentation on human subjects, and suggests that we now appreciate the moral problems posed by animal research roughly as well as we understood those of human experimentation in the late 1960s.[11] This assumes, of course, that animals are generally recognized now as having a kind of moral standing that renders their treatment in our hands problematical; Beauchamp explicitly expresses the hope that we are past the "bad old days" when it was not yet widely acknowledged that animals are morally considerable in their own right.

The "bad old days" are dramatically evoked by an excerpt from the transcript of a panel discussion among eminent animal researchers following the PBS showing of "Primate," a graphic depiction of extremely invasive research. A nonscientist also involved in the post-film discussion, the Harvard philosopher Robert Nozick, suggested that the treatment of the animals in research posed ethical problems because of considerations ultimately having to do with the animals themselves; his interlocutors seemed to find this altogether wrong-headed.[12] Whether we are now, as Beauchamp believes, in a position where Nozick's suggestion would no longer be repudiated, is open to question.

Cora Diamond thinks that there remains an issue about whether the experimental use of animals raises any moral concerns at all, apart, perhaps, from those involved in the efficient use of costly and delicate resources.[13] She has argued with great subtlety that plainly ignoring the moral significance of animal life—as did Nozick's interlocutors, from all appearances—is a moral "cop out."[14] Interaction with animals of the kind that characterizes scientific research blunts our ethical sensibilities. Work of that sort, as she sees it, has a tendency to place us further from the ethical goal of being "people on whom nothing is lost."[15]

Diamond tellingly supports this point by a quotation from a 1912 pamphlet written in support of animal experimentation. The pamphlet details an experimental animal's "great delight" in the appearance of the experimenter who came regularly to examine an induced gastric fistula. The point of the story, from the viewpoint of the anecdote's author, was that the dog not only did not suffer at all, it was actually enthusiastic about its life.

> The dog not only suffered no pain, it also showed great delight—just like a dog that has been sitting about the house, and wants to run out for a walk. When it saw that I was going to look into its stomach, it frisked about in the same way as if I was going to take it out for a walk.[16]

Diamond draws attention to what the defender of research is missing in this story—how pathetic it is that this animal's life should come down to this, that the examination of its stomach is the high point of its existence. The problem with taking research on animals for granted is that it introduces and reinforces a kind of compartmentalization in our responses: what is done in the name of science simply does not raise the kind of moral issues that are raised by similar behavior outside that sphere. The social psychologist will design research proposals that necessitate telling lies, the animal experimenter will structure research that ignores the reality of animal pain and the fact that they are creatures with lives of their own. And this, not as the result of a finely nuanced, vivid conception of the morally problematic nature of what is being done, but rather as a general policy of exempting scientific work from the moral scrutiny to which other kinds of human activity are subject. Diamond's position is powerfully argued. But critics might reply that what it means to achieve has, to a large extent, already occurred; science is no longer considered immune from ethical assessment, and this is particularly true of animal experimentation. But having admitted that such work stands in need of moral assessment, what is to guide that assessment? Granted the ethical significance of a fully realized perception of what one is doing, and of the irresponsibility of ignoring the moral component of one's activity, how are we to balance an imaginative realization of the burden to research animals against an equally empathetic conception of the benefits to humans? What will guide us in choosing between the chimpanzee and the child?

Animals from a Utilitarian Perspective

Most people will regard this as no contest. Animals may have a place in common morality, but it is restricted to a protection against cruel handling, where "cruelty" seems understood as either out-and-out sadism, or, at most, an indifference to the balance of cost and benefit incurred by the infliction of pain or death to animals. Most scientific uses of animals will be untouched by an injunction against cruelty to animals so understood; this will be all the more true for therapeutic uses of animals, as in xenograft. But if such meager protection is all that animals do enjoy from common moral practice, it does not follow that they ought not to get a better deal. The very features on the basis of which animals are accorded any moral standing may entail that they deserve a more secure position. If, for example, we abjure cruelty to animals on the grounds (at least in part) that we believe they can suffer pain, our exclusion of that pain from fair assessment in a utilitarian calculus may seem arbitrary.

Peter Singer's 1975 work, *Animal Liberation*, focused on animal sentience as the fundamental moral analog between humans and members of nonhuman species, arguing that sentience was a necessary and sufficient condition for the possession of interests, and that morality requires, at a minimum, the impartial consideration of all affected interests in the determination of justifiable actions and policies. The "equal consideration of interests" principle was offered as a way of accounting for our intuitions regarding the perniciousness of racism and sexism; this principle explains the sense in which all women and men are equal, without any commitment to kinds of factual equality that may not, as a matter of fact, obtain. They are equal in that their interests deserve fair consideration, regardless of differences of race or gender—even if such differences should turn out to be correlated with differences in certain kinds of abilities. Different types of people may have, as a matter of fact, different types of interests—this is surely true of women and men, for instance—but whatever interests they do have, it is immoral to dismiss or discount them because of biological differences. To do so is to be a racist or a sexist. Precisely the same analysis holds for members of other species. As sentient beings, they have morally considerable interests. Those interests may well be different from—perhaps fewer than—interests possessed by members of the human species. But qua interests, they deserve impartial consideration. If we refuse such consideration, if we discount or dismiss their interests, then we are guilty of speciesism.

Singer's account has had a tremendous impact on the character of philosophical discussion since its publication, and there is evidence that it has had an effect on practice as well. But theoretically, Singer's account is not especially novel. It is simply a consistent working out of act-utilitarian ethics as applied to animals, thus following in the footsteps of one of utilitarianism's progenitors, Jeremy Bentham. About the moral standing of animals, Bentham wrote, "The point is not, Can they reason? nor Can they talk? but, Can they suffer?"[17] If they can—and not many would nowadays follow Descartes in denying it—then they are subjects of moral consideration from a utilitarian perspective.

The common moral tradition affords Singer, and like-minded critics of current practices involving animals, a dialectical foothold, since it accords to animals the sort of direct moral significance referred to above. On this basis, the dismissal or discounting of animal interests can be seen as arbitrary, as the development of the analogy with racism and sexism is designed to illustrate. By far the greater part of Singer's text is devoted to documenting the extent to which animal interests are dismissed in such areas as intensive farming, product testing, and scientific research. Without discussing such difficult questions as how one can compare utilities across species generally, he displays how prevalent is our callousness toward animals. His portrayal of intensive farming practices is particularly powerful and persuasive. Animals are routinely maltreated in much of contemporary "factory farming," and that treatment is difficult to justify by appeal to the benefits incurred. Since human nutritional needs can be tastily satisfied by a vegetarian diet, there would seem to be no fundamental need that can be satisfied only by current practices.

Singer is also extremely critical of animal experimentation, arguing that a great deal of such research is poorly designed, shoddily executed, and aimed at trivial goals. But the issues involving experimentation are crucially different from those involved in agriculture, since the benefits at which researchers aim (even if erratically) are more substantial than certain kinds of gustatory sensations (which would seem to be the only utilities not generally obtainable by a vegetarian diet), and it is unclear that those benefits could be garnered by alternative methods. An illustration of the different kinds of issues involved in animal use in farming and experimentation, respectively, is provided by the difference in the kinds of action to which Singer calls his readers. *Animal Liberation* argues that we have a moral duty to boycott the products of intensive farming, and hence to become vegetarians. But there is no similar call to boycott the products of animal experimentation. We are not urged to use only those medical regimens that have not been tested on animals. This difference in strategy may have been recommended by utilitarian reasoning. Singer may hold that the use of animals in medical research may actually diminish overall utilities, but since we place such importance on our health, calling on people to reject such products would not at all aid in the amelioration of animal suffering; one step at a time may be the practical watchword when trying to uproot certain kinds of pernicious prejudice. But it is more likely that Singer is aware of the significant utilities produced by certain kinds of animal experimentation, and that his position here is at base reformist, rather than revolutionary.

The extent of the reform ought not to be minimized; as a measure of our good faith in proposing the use of an animal in medical or other experimentation (or, one presumes, therapy) on the grounds that the benefits at large outweigh the costs to the individual animals, Singer suggests that we consider whether we would be willing to subject a "marginal" human being to the same experiment. Would we, that is, be willing to experiment upon a human being who, in all morally relevant respects, is identical to an animal? Say, a human being who was mentally retarded and an orphan, capable of no more intellection, relativity, or personality than the primates who would be the alternative candidates for the procedure? For if we are not so willing, then we are not impartially weighing the burdens and benefits of the proposed research. Rather, we are allowing a bias toward members of our own species to creep in.

The logic of this move is interesting. Other writers—in particular, Tom Regan[18]—have used similar considerations in support of an account of animal moral standing that ascribes to them not merely the right to equal consideration of interests—which is actually not so much a right as a statement of their inclusion in the utilitarian calculus—but rather a right to life, as well as to freedom from the infliction of nontrivial and unwarranted pain, and to respectful treatment. This is a much more ambitious use of the argument, and will be examined at some length below. But even in Singer's hands, the argument invites scrutiny. The argument was first met with attempts to specify properties held by "marginal" humans that were not possessed by animals, and that were also morally relevant. R. G. Frey, perhaps the most prominent act-utilitarian to oppose "animal liberation," sympathetically surveyed some likely candidates—that some humans put in the marginal class had morally significant potentials lacked by animals supposedly on a par with them; that humans may possess, whereas animals

may lack, "souls," and that there are morphological similarities between paradigmatic and marginal humans that are greater than
those between humans and comparison animals.[19] As Frey later
came to admit, none of these considerations are decisive.[20] Other
philosophers have also attempted to discern morally relevant
differences; one attempt in particular will be discussed later in this
chapter.

Interestingly enough, some writers—including Frey—are now
taking a different tack on this question, and are arguing that the
"marginal cases argument" succeeds not in elevating the status of
animals, but in revealing that the moral status of profoundly retarded human orphans is lower than we have assumed, and that such
humans ought in principle to be equally eligible for nonconsensual,
painful and/or lethal research. In a recent issue of the *Journal of
Medical Ethics*, Thomasine Kushner and Raymond Belliotti argue
that anencephalic neonates be used as sources of organs in preference to animals. They even envisage a colony of massively
retarded humans kept in readiness for organ donation, thus troping
suggestions made by xenograft researchers in the past that colonies
of primates be maintained for the express purpose of xenograft donations.[21]

The implications of this shift of emphasis will be explored below. At this point, I want to examine other aspects of Singer's use
of the marginal cases argument. Although it can be understood in
a purely *ad hominem*, rhetorical fashion, I believe Singer actually
does see the properties typically possessed by members of the
human species to be of particular moral value, for they are the basis
for the possession of interests that go beyond those typically possessed by nonhuman animals. If the goal of the moral life is to
maximize the satisfaction of interests, then since typical humans—
or "persons"—are richer generators of interests, they can be regarded as morally more significant without transgressing the equal
consideration of interests principle, without incurring speciesism.
This feature of the utilitarian case for the elevation of animal moral
status has serious implications for the critique of animal experi-

mentation, and for the therapeutic use of animals in particular. If persons are such that utility can generally be maximized by preserving and extending their lives over those of other organisms with a less extensive range of interests, and if the utilization of animals in research and therapy is a uniquely significant way of securing this benefit, then it would seem that at least many medical employments of animals could go on, provided that any discomfort suffered by the animals was taken seriously and reduced insofar as is consistent with optimal utilities.

In the absence of any demonstrable distinction between animals and marginal human beings, we might have to adopt the proposals urged recently by Frey and by Kushner and Belliotti. But even if no "intrinsic" morally significant difference between the species could be uncovered, surely utilitarians would have to be sensitive to such "side effects" as the revulsion many people would experience at the prospect of such experimental and therapeutic uses of infants and others, and, in any event, it is not yet established that there are no such differences.

Other writers have tried to demonstrate the existence among animals of richer moral analogs to persons than merely our shared sentience. Two of the most notable attempts have been made by Regan, in his work *The Case for Animal Rights*, and in a series of articles by Steven F. Sapontzis.[22] Regan's rights-based approach has somewhat less ambiguous implications for the use of animals in experimentation and therapy than does Singer's; outside, perhaps, of those ways in which we would consent to the use of children in medical research, the utilization of nonhumans in experimentation and therapy is apparently morally excluded.

Animals as Holders of Moral Rights

In the initial development of his view, Regan relied heavily on the argument from marginal cases, holding that, since we ascribe the right to life and to freedom from suffering to damaged human beings who in all morally relevant respects are identical to many nonhumans, we must, if we are to be consistent, assign the same rights to the comparable nonhumans. Many animals—including many of those we eat and experiment upon—are, in Regan's terminology, "subjects of a life," a life whose value is to be determined independently of its usefulness to others. It is in recognition of the intrinsic value of their lives that we are prepared to honor damaged humans by extending them the right to life and to freedom from suffering, and it is in virtue of precisely the same feature of animal lives that we ought to assign to them the same moral respects. Animals, like human beings, are Kantian moral persons, ends in themselves, rather than means to another's ends, although they do not enjoy this status in virtue of their ratiocinative abilities.

Some of the recent responses to the marginal cases argument surveyed above may suggest problems with this line of approach, and may also explain why Regan's most comprehensive statement, *The Case for Animal Rights*, does not rely heavily on the analogies between retarded persons and animals. Frey's call for possibly lethal and painful experimentation on retarded children, and Belliotti and Kushner's planned colony of marginal human organ donors, may suggest that drawing attention to the similarities between animals and certain human beings has more the effect of diminishing the status of the latter than of enhancing that of the former. Moreover, the general questions in medical ethics concerning the status of damaged neonates may seem to indicate a much shakier consenus in moral intuition regarding the status of such beings than Regan assumes.

Actually, this line of criticism may be less formidable than it appears. Frey's view is, I think, idiosyncratic, and misses a certain kind of moral disanalogy between animals and marginal humans that, while not undermining Regan's argument, does provide a way of distinguishing between them for the purpose of determining who—if anyone—might be a legitimate research subject. What Frey has missed is the significance of our emotional response to the birth of a massively damaged child or to the reduction to "marginal" status of a formerly "paradigmatic" person. We feel such happenings to be tragic. On the other hand, the birth of a healthy animal, on a psychological par with the retarded human, does not, in itself, constitute a tragedy at all.

Our response in such cases is not simply a matter of emotional prejudice; it is not emotional speciesism that leads us to feel this way. Our feeling is based on a significant difference in the cases: a marginal human has suffered a loss of tragic proportions. It makes perfect sense to think about the kind of life that human might have had, to feel pity and compassion with her or him over the loss, and, in token of respect for that loss, to refuse to add to the burdens of an already tragically affected being. The animal which, in all morally significant factual respects, is identical to the human, is not identical in all the morally relevant counterfactual respects.[23]

With respect to the Kushner-Belliotti discussion, their serious recommendation is actually focused on anencephalic humans. Anencephaly is a condition incompatible with life, and even if this were not the case, it is arguable that such humans fall below the level occupied in general by many animals, and hence that what is morally appropriate respecting their treatment is not significantly informative regarding animals. Of course, it is arguable that the anencephalics have suffered a particularly massive tragedy, and that their situation deserves our pity and compassion as well. But the position here is not that the proper response to someone who has undergone such a tragedy is that they never be used as subjects of research, or as organ donors, but rather that we place on them no more burdens than we can help; it is not clear that the Kushner-Belliotti suggestion is actually burdensome to anencephalics. A good deal of the philosophical debate over the appropriate treatment of damaged neonates is not directly a discussion about what kind of attention is owing to them morally. Rather, it is a debate about what it is to scrupulously care for the interests of such patients, about what respecting them as persons may actually entail in tragic circumstances.

These last remarks have been an attempt to indicate that the line of argument that characterized Regan's "early" work is still worthy of attention. Regan now still relies heavily on the notion of animals (in particular, mammals of a year of age or more) as "subjects of a life," and still regards them as properly included in the class of those whose lives and comfort are protected by morality. Regan argues that, although some animals apparently lack consciousness, and others, although conscious and sentient, lack beliefs, many fully meet the requirements for having a life of their own. Their behavior is best explained by attributing to them beliefs, desires, and a self-concept, a temporal awareness, and a kind of autonomy Regan calls "preference autonomy," which refers to an animal's ability to act according to its own preferences.

Creatures who possess traits of this kind possess a welfare; that is, their lives can be better or worse for them, from their own subjective standpoint. The value of their existence is not wholly a matter of their usefulness as instruments to others' ends. Nonhumans of this sort, as well as humans, possess inherent value, and on Regan's view, the possession of inherent value is a categorical matter: it is not the case that, of a plurality of beings all enjoying intrinsic value, some do so to a greater degree than others.

A chief support for attributing intrinsic value categorically comes from a rejection of "perfectionist" moralities, i. e., theories that make moral standing a variable matter, with the variation determined by how one scores on an appropriate scale: intelligence, or virtue, say. If we want to say that human subjects of a life matter more than animal subjects of a life, we are logically committed to making the extent to which one enjoys such traits as intelligence to be strongly relevant to moral status. Regan regards such a position as repugnant to nonaristocratic moral intuitions, and, in an interesting and valuable section of the book, provides a mechanism for sorting out morally valid from morally suspect intuitions.

Regan's position is also marked by a strong critique of utilitarianism, which, in his view, has implications that outrage properly formed moral intuitions. He believes—and in this makes common cause with Frey—that including animals within a utilitarian calculus will not call for substantial alteration in the ways in which we treat animals—at least, it has not been shown by utilitarian animal advocates like Singer that the overall utility will be improved by major changes. Comparatively minor reforms of meat production and research techniques would probably satisfy the calculus of utility.

Regan's "rights view" holds that all members of the moral community—i.e., both moral agents, such as human persons, and moral patients, such as the nonhumans he focuses upon—possess a set of basic rights that they enjoy independently of their activities or relationships. These rights are distributed universally and are held equally strongly among the members of the entire community. They include a right to respectful treatment, which forbids regarding an individual as if he or she were a mere receptacle of value, as utilitarianism would imply; it insists that individuals have intrinsic moral value. All moral agents and patients also have a *prima facie* right not to be harmed by others.

An extensive challenge to Regan's view is presented by Michael A. Fox in his recent *Case for Animal Experimentation*.[24] Fox denies that animals are sufficiently well equipped psychologically to make judgments about their own welfare, and hence that they cannot be held to have an intrinsic value. But he also offers an internal critique of the notion that animals have other than instrumental value. Animal intrinsic value must be either (1) equal to that of human persons (as Regan maintains) or (2) less that than of human persons (as Singer maintains). But the former view would seem to forbid our sacrificing animal interests to any human need (since animals are always innocent of wrongdoing and can never consent to their utilization) and this is massively counterintuitive. The latter view is unstable; it collapses with Singer's willingness to prefer humans to animals in situations where human life is at stake.[25]

These arguments of Fox's seem ill-considered. A utilitarian willingness to use one being as a means to another's ends does not entail a denial that the creature being used has intrinsic value; it is simply that the optimum amount of intrinsic value is producible only through that sacrifice. And Regan holds, plausibly enough, that two creatures can each have equal intrinsic value, but can face situations that constitute unequal harms to them. In such cases, we are not forbidden by our respect for their equal intrinsic value from treating them unequally. Typically, Regan claims, death will be a greater harm to human subjects-of-a-life than to animal subjects, and we are acting properly if we save such a person over an animal. This position might seem to leave a large loophole for certain types of animal experiments to continue and to pave the way to the ethical acceptablility of xenograft in particular. But in fact it does not. We are not allowed to use some animal's death to secure a person's life, even though death is a greater harm to the person than to the animal. That involves using the animal as a means to the person's ends, which is incompatible with the respect owed to subjects of a life. However, if we are facing a situation in which we must choose to save the life of a person or the life of an animal—a lifeboat sort of case—we may choose to save the "worse off" of the two, the human.

A more significant loophole concerns the use of animals who are not "subjects of a life." Regan's chief concern in *The Case for Animal Rights* is with mammals of one year of age or greater; such animals, he argues, clearly possess the psychological capacities to render them subjects of a life, with an inherent value that morality must respect. A great deal of experimentation is done on nonmammalian animals and on animals younger than one year old. So it seems that even procedures that typically involve "higher" animals—such as xenograft—could go on consistently with the rights view, as long as the animals involved are young enough. (In his communication in the *Journal of the American Medical Association*, Dr. Leonard Bailey, the surgeon in the Baby Fae case, and his coworkers, speak of the baboon donors as "young," and in the informed consent document for that operation, the animal is referred to as "immature."[26]

Regan, however, replies to such possibilities that the status of subject of a life, although sufficient for the possession of rights, is not necessary, and further cautions us to be careful of the psychological effects of using immature and nonmammalian animals in research (as well as in other contexts). What Regan is apparently offering, then, is a two-tiered system of animal ethics: adult mammals are protected by "direct duties" we have to them in virtue of their status as subjects of a life; other animals are protected by "indirect duties" we have to them via our duties to other animals and to humans, as well as by the prudential consideration that we are not sure that such creatures do not have at least some rights inhering in their own person. Especially given Regan's own criticism of indirect duty views in point of their arbitrariness,[27] this aspect of his view seems weak. Perhaps Regan should relax his opposition to utilitarianism, at least to the point of accepting a "rights for subjects of a life, utilitarianism for sentient nonsubjects of a life" position if he is to provide any kind of moral protection to, say, the billions of chickens that are intensively reared and consumed in the US, and the tens of thousands of rats and mice that are subject to painful experimentation.

A position more eclectic in its defense of animals has been developed by Steven F. Sapontzis. Sapontzis finds in animals analogs to human experience that engage many elements of common morality. Animals are not only sentient, and hence worthy of consideration insofar as the moral life involving maximizing the satisfaction of interests; they are not only subjects of a life, and hence deserving of whatever moral regard is due such creatures; they are also, in many instances, virtuous beings, who deserve the respect we tender to those whose lives exemplify traits of character we regard as morally admirable.

Making a case for animal virtue, and a case for the significance of the virtues in our assessments, occupies Sapontzis in a series of recent articles.[28] Sapontzis highlights the extent to which moral standing ought to be considered not a matter following from the possession of certain properties, but rather a matter of the moral character of the individual in question. That animals—at least, many animals—have the traits that are necessary for the expression of virtues may seem doubtful. But the rational support for such doubt stems from features of philosophical ethics rather remote from "common sense morality." For example, the Kantian kind of view, which would make rationality and the execution of the moral law for the law's own sake necessary for morally admirable action, is belied by our tendency to think better of the father who loves his children out of inclination than we do of the father whose love is a matter of duty. On Sapontzis's analysis, the parental affection, courage, friendship, ingenuity, loyalty, and so on that we ascribe to animals ought to be understood just as we understand the corresponding virtues in humans, and redound equally to the credit of nonhuman virtuous beings as to human. Nothing in the differences between humans and nonhumans is sufficient to rob virtuous behavior of its moral merit. Like Regan, Sapontzis's position is much more revolutionary than reformist when it comes to considering the ethical status of animal experimentation. Although some types of nonintrusive research could go on, the great majority of scientific intervention into the lives of animals is wrong and ought to stop. Both Regan[29] and Sapontzis[30] have explicitly written against the use of animals in xenograft. But, because of its theoretical eclecticism (which is itself a consequence of Sapontzis's interest in and respect for the resources of common morality), his position may provide a more thoroughgoing critique of a wider range of animal experimentation that does that of Regan.

It is arguable, however, that Regan's views constitute a further impediment to animal research of even the nonintrusive kind. Consider that the justification for insisting on informed consent in experimentation is, at least to deontologically oriented theorists, not so much a matter of subject protection as it is a token of respect for the persons involved. They are not to be seen as means to the researcher's ends solely, and their consent is sought as a means of securing that end. Some writers have argued that, from such a deontological perspective, even nonintrusive research needs to satisfy the requirement of consent.[31] Regan's position is, of course, highly deontological, and, although he has not written explicitly about the moral underpinnings of the informed consent requirement, it seems reasonable to believe that he would regard that requirement in a nonconsequentialist light.

Since mammals of one year of age or more are moral persons (even if not necessarily moral agents), then it would seem that certain kinds of noninvasive, observational research on animals might still be seen as using them as means to our ends, and hence as wrong. Animals might well be seen best as we see children, and hence as drawn into all the kinds of problems that beset us when we consider pediatric experimentation, even in "no-risk" contexts.[32]

Xenograft and Partial Affections

Positions such as those surveyed above tend to respond to the issue of xenograft rather categorically. Despite some worries about what the letter of Regan's text implies for young animals, it seems to follow from his and from Sapontzis's theories (and certainly from their own accounts of the matter) that xenograft is to be forbidden; Frey and Fox and (perhaps surprisingly) Singer would permit it, at least as far as issues concerning the moral status of animals are concerned. This may be too general an approach to a difficult problem.

In an earlier paper,[33] I explored the possibility that parents of children who are candidates for lifesaving xenograft (assuming that there were such a thing) are in a significantly different position ethically from scientists and physicians choosing to engage in research aimed at the development of xenotransplantation as a usable therapy. In brief, the argument of that paper is that considerations of impartial moral reason do not support regarding animals as spare parts bins for humans; this is an especially weighty consideration when one keeps in mind the characteristics of the species that are the prime candidates for the role of donor in xenotransplantation. There seems little question that primates such as Goobers, the baboon who "donated" her heart for Baby Fae, possess traits that are strongly morally analogous to those possessed by our paradigm exemplars of morally considerable beings, human persons. Goobers was not only sentient; she had a life of her own, one potentially richer than many granted to human beings. In the absence of theological considerations (whose role in the determination of public policy remains problematic), it seems that Regan and Sapontzis, and all those who would draw our attention to the ways in which such animals as Goobers may be harmed, and to the reasons for which inflicting such harm is incompatible with the role such beings ought to have in our moral community, are correct: such animals ought not to be viewed as unwilling sources of human transplant organs.

But there is another side to the story, another audience for the question, "Is xenograft moral?" than the medical researcher's. Parents, and those who stand in the place of parents, may find themselves with a child with a congenital heart defect such as the HLHS that confronted Baby Fae. Was it wrong for Fae's parents to consent to her xenograft? Would it be wrong for future parents facing a similar problem to consent to refined versions of such therapy?

These two questions may be importantly different: the issues that faced Fae's parents included, surely, whether the proposed intervention was even in Fae's interests. In their report on the site visit to Loma Linda University, where Fae's surgery took place, the NIH team expressed concern over the extent to which the involved physicians stressed the possibilities of long-term survival for Fae, possibilities that struck the team as being extremely remote. It may well have been the case that there were two experimental animals in this situation, both Goobers and Fae, and that the role of each in this operation was to benefit others than themselves. If so, there are surely questions about the permissibility of exposing Fae to the morbidity involved in the transplant procedure; if cadaver organs were truly unavailable and the other possible surgical procedure seemed to hold out no significant hope for survival, what we may have owed to Fae was to ease, rather than burden, her dying.

But if the xenographic procedure had actually been of real and unique therapeutic value—if it and no other therapy held out a realistic chance for Fae's survival—it seems to me that a strong case can be made for the permissibility of her parent's decision. I do not mean that their decision would be forgivable in the light of the extreme pressure they faced. I am asserting, rather, that the partiality that such parents have toward their children is morally admirable, and that it legitimates, at least if certain other conditions are met, the use of a nonhuman primate's heart (or other vital organ) in order to keep that child alive (at least, if life is truly in that child's interest).

This is a position that is likely to please no one. Proponents of enhancing the moral status of animals will likely see in my claim that parents can offer their children something vital to the survival of an animal, a speciesism occluded by sentimentality; those who are unconvinced by the arguments of Regan, Sapontzis, et al., will think that the position needs no justification insofar as the child's parents are concerned, but then will reject the limitation in the scope of this proposal: parents, yes; researchers, no.

Can one consistently hold that moral principles—impartial moral reason—indict xenograft, whereas parental relationships—partial affections—provide a context in which those moral principles may be waived? Does this not conflict with the universality of moral principles?

It seems to me that there are two ways of responding to this. One would be to say that parental duties are merely "local instances" of general duties of, say, utility maximization or fairness, and for reasons still to be developed, I am holding that parental duties outweigh the duties of more general scope. But this is surely compatible with allowing the universality of moral principle.

The second possible response would be to hold that the kinds of moral considerations that range over parents here are not like general duties, that what we have here is a clash between two kinds of morally significant notions: moral principles and moral affection. This would seem the less promising line to pursue. In fact, insofar as I want to argue that all parents (and all those who stand in the position of parents to children) ought to resolve the dilemma this way, it seems that I am willy-nilly establishing it as a moral principle that conflicts between parental duties and general duties ought in such cases be resolved in favor of the former. However, I think that regarding this situation as altogether and simply a clash between duties will obscure certain features of the parent-child relationship.

What is morally owing to children from parents? In large part, what is owed is the sense that the child is not simply another morally considerable being whose autonomy I must respect, whose interests I must impartially weigh, whose virtues I must respect. Rather, children need—and deserve—to be singled out as special recipients of the care and affection of their parents. Some part of the normativity of this relationship may be explained by considerations of reciprocity among generations: my parents acted so to me, now I must carry on the tradition, and give the same gift to my children. Some part may be explained in terms of considerations of the overall utility; I may favor my children over other claimants of the benefits I might provide because so arranging the disposition of the care of children results in the most favorable ratio of good over evil. But I am doubtful that these considerations exhaust the moral character of the relations between parents and children. Would my obligations to my children differ had I not been loved by my parents? Is it clear that parental particularism is in fact optimific from a utilitarian perspective?

What children need to find in their relationship with their parents is not solely impartial respect, but intense partial affection (which does not exclude an appreciation of the child's general moral status). This affection will issue forth in actions and dispositions of a sort that may be consistent with what is owing to children from the perspective of impartial moral reason, but those actions are not motivated by such considerations, at least not generally. And the love itself—which is not an agapeistic love, but rather a love that is by its nature preferential—is not something that can be commanded. Like nonagapeistic love generally, it is best regarded as a gift, not as the result of performing a duty. But the character of those who give or who withhold such a gift is subject to moral assessment; it is part of being a virtuous parent to give this gift to one's children; it is a vice in parents to withhold it.

In his recent work, *Parents & Children: The Ethics of the Family,* Jeffrey Blustein says that to speak, as he does, of the nature and source of parental obligation is not to deny the importance—perhaps even the greater importance—of those parts of being a good parent that do not reduce to talk of duties.[34] In developing his theory of familial duties, he wishes only to provide a guide to how natural affection should express itself, as well as a set of concerns that should bolster our tendencies to act well toward our children during those periods when we might be inclined otherwise. This is surely a valid concern, but it is not clear that it is necessary to talk of moral duties—if those are thought to be moral norms established independently of the love that good parents bear their children—in order to address it. For if what is morally fundamental about the parent–child relationship stems from the application of general moral norms to respect persons and promote utility then the status of the relationship is derivative, and could in principle be altered. And the argumentative strategy raises questions here as well: if the point of introducing talk of duties is to bolster backsliding parents, is it likely to be more useful than other kinds of exhortations, which might focus not on duties, but on the children and the relationship?

Later, Blustein grapples with the issue of whether the existence of the family is consistent with our social commitment to providing equal opportunity. Quite a fair case can be made that it is not, and that both the deontological and the consequentialist values that would be served by observation of this principle are not being enhanced by the maintenance of strong, particularistic family structures. But we tend to feel, I think, that such considerations, even if successful, do not make the case against the family; there are values residing there that are important independently of their relationship to general moral norms and empirical conditions. If our society would, in the long run, be only marginally happier, only marginally fairer for the abandonment of the kinds of intimate partialities that undergird the family, I believe that we would not hurry to alter matters, and that it would be more than mere inertia that would cause us to hesitate.

So it seems to me that there are morally respectable considerations that are rooted in the nature of what it is to be a virtuous parent, which make the conflict between someone like Baby Fae and someone like Goobers more than simply a dilemma of character. It is not something that needs only an appreciation of the relevant moral principles and empirical considerations, along with the courage of one's convictions, to resolve. It is, rather, a dilemma of values: impartial moral norms make extremely problematic the use of (at least some) animals as sources of vital organs for persons, whereas the virtues appropriate to being a good parent may, in relevant circumstances, make it obligatory to accept the offer of xenograft.

But even if I am correct in suggesting that there may well be a real moral dilemma here, what supports the resolution I suggest, and what are the implications of that resolution? The most significant support I can offer for this particular resolution is that it is a way of keeping faith with more of the morally relevant circumstances occasioned by the case—or, at least, it can be. If, out of respect for the moral significance of the life of the animal, parents should reject the offer of xenotransplantation in those circumstances in which it would be necessary to save a child's life, the parents have elected to respect "impartial" moral considerations at the expense of partial ones. If, on the other hand, the parents accept the offer, they can choose other means to express their respect for those impartial moral norms. They can, for example, work against the extension of the use of animals in medical therapy and experimentation, thus adopting a version of the "concerned individual" strategy that R. G. Frey has offered as an acceptable response to the moral problems involved in the intensive rearing of animals for food.[35]

This suggestion raises consistency problems; can a person accept the benefits of a procedure, while at the same time campaigning actively against it? In other words, parents who try to strike a balance between the competing values here involved seem to be willing to use for the benefit of their own child that which they will deny to the children of others—if not present children, then to future children, living at a time when (as the animal advocate hopes) animal organs are no longer harvested from living donors for human needs.

What makes all this even more problematic is that this issue occurs not only in the case of xenotransplantation. People sensitive to the moral claims of animals face in the entire medical establishment a host of procedures and agents that are of real value, but that at the same time are the result of immense amounts of animal suffering. If we conclude that such people cannot consistently avail themselves of the benefits of xenotransplantation—or make it available to their children—what other restrictions follow? Pro-animal activists and theorists have repeatedly advocated abstention from animal products in the categories of food and clothing; should such abstention be extended to the categories of medicine and health care as well? Surely, the values conflicting with respectful treatment of animals are weightier in the medical sphere, and this should make a difference to those who approach these questions from a strictly utilitarian basis. But for those like Regan and Sapontzis, who attribute to animals a right to life and respectful treatment, the issue is more difficult.

Yet if a virtuous parent/concerned individual strategy is appropriate for xenotransplantation, and other therapies exploitative of animals, and if animal moral status is best understood in terms of their possessing rights, will it not follow that the combination of need, virtuous disposition, and respect for general moral norms that characterizes this strategy also legitimates the use of human persons in such ways? And if the answer to this question is "no," will that not indicate that humans are (in general) of more significance than nonhumans? The implication of that would seem to be that xenograft, and related uses of animals, would be justified on general moral grounds. The appeal to special parental responsibilities and to the moral legitimacy of partial affections would, in that case, be quite beside the point.[36]

I think the best response here follows Regan in admitting that the death of a person is typically a greater harm than it is to a nonhuman, and yet maintains that this does not allow the sacrifice of the animal to a person's interest in general, although Regan does take it to justify the choice of a human over a nonhuman in cases in which they are in a direct "overcrowded lifeboat" style of conflict. But this does not imply that animals may be used as means to human ends generally, nor does it explain why humans to whom death is not a greater harm than it is to animals should be in any protected position. Would a parent situated as I have described have the right to accept the offer of a marginal human being's vital organ?

I would at this point again appeal to the tragic character of the circumstances of such humans, and would maintain that we ought not to be the sort of people who are insensitive to the harm already suffered by such humans. If, in order to save the life of a child, a parent must accept an organ "donated" by either an animal or a psychologically equivalent human, one is not being arbitrary if one selects the organ from the nonhuman. The animal has not suffered the same kind of loss that the human has, and hence is not, in that respect, a proper subject of the pity and compassion of the parent. This, of course, does not settle the question of whether a virtuous parent/concerned individual could accept an ill-gotten organ from a marginal human if there were no animal alternatives, but it does indicate the existence of another moral constraint, lack-ing in animal cases, that the parent's duties would have to override. I am inclined to think, for this and other reasons, that parents ought not to accept an organ stolen from a marginal human (at least, if the theft were of something that had value to the human); the situation with, say, anencephalic infants may be different.

Conclusion

The progress of modern medicine is tightly wrapped up with the use of animals; the advent of xenotransplantation simply intensifies that relationship. There are, as mentioned above, many reasons to welcome the further contributions animals may come to make to our health. Yet at the same time, as scientists have been discerning and employing deep physical analogies between humans and other animals, other scholars have been exploring the moral analogies that exist between the species, and finding them to be surprisingly deep as well. These moral analogies—for example, sentience, being the subject of a life, being virtuous—cast into doubt our right to exploit the physical similarities among us as blithely as we have done, and call into question the moral legitimacy of xenograft, and indeed, the whole enterprise of medical research as it is presently constituted.

Similar points effectively undermine the licitness of factory farming, as well as others of the myriad ways in which we use animals as means to our ends solely, with little or no regard for the animals as such. But the medical context is an extremely complicated one. Unlike other ways in which we use animals, the services presented in medicine and health care are extraordinarily important to our vital interests, and are deeply bound up with our ideals of what it is to appropriately care for ourselves and others—in particular, to those whose care is especially our responsibility. Refusing such people the benefits of the present health care system—benefits that, for all the many ways in which they may be ethically problematic are often essential for life and for fulfilling life—is itself extraordinarily problematic.

In my judgment, we ought not to attempt to solve the moral problems of allocation involved in organ transplant by the use of animals. We ought rather to seek out ways to tap the community's altruism more deeply and to more efficiently employ available human resources than we do at present. But this recommendation only pushes the underlying problem back a step. The moral burden that our current orientation in medicine incurs from its use of animals is still another reason to consider changing that orientation to one more involved with prevention than cure, one less dependent on cost-ineffective, fundamentally inegalitarian technological solutions, to one more dependent on the assumption of personal responsibility for health and for the dangerous behaviors with which we make ourselves more likely candidates for batteries of treatment whose cost exceeds the economic.[37]

Notes and References

[1]For and overview of technical and ethical issues in organ transplantation, see *Organ Transplantation: Issues and Recommendations*, the Report of the Task Force on Organ Transplantation (US Department of Health and Human Services, April, 1986).

[2]Arthur L. Caplan "Ethical Issues Raised by Research Involving Xenografts," *JAMA* **254** (23), 1985, p. 3340.

[3]See the report of the Council on Scientific Affairs, "Xenograft: Review of the Literature and Current Status" in *JAMA* **254** (23), 1985, p. 3354.

[4]The development of the new immunosuppressants have led some experts to question the extent to which donor–recipient compatability is any longer a crucial issue in transplantation success. *See* J. F. Childress, "Organ Transplantation," *Bioethics Reporter* (1986).

[5]For cardiac xenograft preceding Baby Fae's, see the reports by J. D. Hardy, et al., "Heart Transplantation in Man," *JAMA* **198**, 1964, pp. 114-122 and C. N. Bernard et al., "Heterotopic Cardiac Transplantation with a Xenograft for Assitance of the Left Heart in Cardiogenic Shock after Cardiopulmonary Bypass," *South African Medical Journal* **52**, 1977, pp. 1035–1038; for renal xenograft, *see* the report of K. Reemtsma, et al., "Renal Heterotransplantation in Man," *Annals of Surgery* **160**, 1964, pp. 384–408.

[6]*Time*, Nov. 12, 1984, p. 72.

[7]L. Bailey et al. "Baboon-to-Human Cardiac Xenotransplantation in a Neonate." *JAMA* **254** (23), 1985, p. 3321.

[8]"The Subject is Baby Fae," *Hastings Center Report* **15**, 1985.

[9]Microallocation and economic questions are also noted by James F. Childress, in his article "Organ Transplantation," *Bioethics Reporter* (1986). See sections 13-5.1 and 13-5.2.

[10]An indication that this premise is still pretty deeply underground is provided by the "Report of the National Institutes of Health Site Visit to Loma Linda University Medical Center for Purposes of Consultation and Review of Institutional Review Board Procedures in Connection with Cardiac Xenograft Transplantation Program," dated March 5, 1985. This report does not even raise the issue of the moral status of the xenograft donor.

[11]Tom L. Beauchamp, "Problems in Justifying Research on Animals," a rough draft of a paper to be published by the National Academy of Sciences, p. 2.

[12]Ibid., pp. 4–6.

[13]Cora Diamond, "Experimenting with Animals: A Problem in Ethics," in David Sperlinger (ed.), *Animals in Research* (Chichester/New York: John Wiley & Sons, 1981), pp. 338–362.

[14]Ibid., p. 362.

[15]The phrase is taken from Nussbaum's discussion of James' moral project in *The Golden Bowl*. See her "Finely Aware and Richly Responsible: Henry James and the Moral Task of Literature," *Journal of Philosophy* **82** (10), 1985.

[16]Diamond, "Experimenting with Animals," p. 353.

[17]Jeremy Bentham, Introduction to the *Principles of Morals and Legislation*, ch. 18, sec. 1, note.

[18]See, for example, Regan's "An Analysis and Defense of One Argument Concerning Animal Rights," *Inquiry* **22** (1–2), 1979.

[19]R. G. Frey (1982) *Interests and Rights: The Case Against Animals* (Oxford: Clarendon Press), pp. 31–32.

[20]R. G. Frey (1984) *Rights, Killing and Suffering* (Oxford: Basil Blackwell, pp. 113–116). For a fuller consideration of this texts, *see* my "Critical Notice," *Between the Species* **2** (2), 1986.

[21]Thomasine Kushner and Raymond Belliotti "Baby Fae: A Beastly Business," *Journal of Medical Ethics* **11**, 1985. The suggestions concerning maintaining colonies of primate donors were made and discussed in the December 1970 issue of *Transplantation Proceedings* (2,4), which was devoted to cross-species transplantation. See the "Discussion" section on p. 554.

[22]Tom Regan (1983) *The Case for Animal Rights* (Berkeley and Los Angeles, The University of California Press). Representative articles by Steve F. Sapontzis include "Are Animals Moral Beings?" *American Philosophical Quarterly* **17** (1980), "A Critique of Personhood," *Ethics* **91** (1981), and "Moral Value and Reason," *Monist* **66** (1983).

[23]For further discussion of this point, see my "The Tragedy of Marginal Cases," Pacific Division APA, March 1985.

[24]Michael A. Fox (1985) *The Case for Animal Experimentation* (Berkeley and Los Angeles: University of California Press).

[25]Ibid., pp. 88–89.

[26]Bailey et al., 3322. The informed consent document is appended to the "Report of the National Institutes of Health Site Visit."

[27]Regan, *Case for Animal Rights*, p. 185–93.

[28]See note 22.

[29]Regan, "The Subject is Baby Fae," *Hastings Center Report* 15, 1985.

[30]Sapontzis, "Reply to Nelson" in *Between the Species*, 2 (3), 1986.

[31]For a discussion of various ethical "models" undergirding the informed consent requirement, *see* James F. Childress, *Priorities in Biomedical Ethics* (Philadelphia: The Westminister Press, 1981), 3, "Human Subjects in Research."

[32]A classic discussion of these issues is contained in the debate between Ramsey and McCormick; an accessible source is Mappes and Zembaty (eds.) *Abiomedical Ethics* (New York: McGraw-Hill, 1986), pp. 193–205.

[33]James Nelson, "Xenograft and Partial Affection," *Between the Species*, 2 (3), 1986

[34]Jeffrey Blustein (1982) *Parents and Children: The Ethics of the Family* (Oxford: Oxford University Press).

[35]R. G. Frey, *Rights, Killing and Suffering*, ch. 16.

[36]See William Aikens, "Reply to Nelson" in *Between the Species*, 2 (3), 1986.

[37]A good bit of this essay was prepared during Prof. James F. Childress' 1986 NEH Summer Seminar, "Principles and Metaphors in Bioethics." I am grateful to Prof. Childress, and to my colleagues in the seminar, for their contributions to my understanding of some of the issues involved here, as well as to the Endowment for its support of the Summer Seminar Program. I am also very grateful to Ms. Hilde Lindemann Nelson for her philosophical and editorial observations.

The Nurse's Role

Rights and Responsibilities

Introduction

One of the major changes in the health care system in recent decades has been the increased professional responsibility assumed by nurses. The view of nurses as merely executors of the physician's will has been radically challenged by nurses who have tried to define and articulate their own domain of authority within the health care system. One aspect of this change is increased concern by nurses with the ethical principles governing their practice. The pair of papers in this section deals with two aspects of this growing concern with the ethical principles governing nursing.

Marsha D.M. Fowler's paper, "The Nurse's Role: Responsibilities and Rights," is a theoretical examination of the correlative responsibilities and rights of nurses. On the basis of an examination of the moral responsibilities nurses assume, she analyzes the rights nurses require if they are to execute their responsibilities. She begins with a discussion of nursing responsibility, which she construes generally as a matter of advocacy for the patient. She describes four contemporary views of what nurse advocacy entails: advocacy for a patient's legal rights within the health care system, advocacy for the patient's values through helping the patient to clarify and act on those values, advocacy for patient dignity and welfare, and finally, advocacy through protest on behalf of the patient. Without settling on which of these views of advocacy is correct, Fowler turns to the question of what rights nurses need in order to serve their advocate role. First, she contends that nurses require the basic right to protection from reprisal for advocacy actions. Second, they need the right to institutional processes and procedures through which advocacy is possible. In this regard, Fowler discusses both more traditional procedures of appealing upward within the health care hierarchy, and more experimental procedures that utilize institutional ethics committees not only in a judicial manner, but in a quasilegislative way to address recurring problems nurse advocates confront.

Darlene Aulds Martin's article, "The Legacy of Baby Doe: Nurses' Ethical and Legal Obligations to Severely Handicapped Newborns," takes a much more concrete perspective, examining the nurse's responsibility in treatment of severly handicapped newborns. She reviews the general ethical debate that has occurred during the past decade over when, if ever, it is proper to withhold treatment from those who are severly handicapped and allow them to die. She espouses a "best interest" principle that would allow letting these children die only when it is in their best interest, but she also discusses the practical problems in assessing the infant's best interest. After reviewing the checkered history of attempts to bring this assessment before civil bodies, Martin explores what role the nurse could play in these decisions. She argues that the nurse has a special warrant for advocacy on behalf of the severely handicapped child since the nurse is the principal healer and surrogate mother, and introduces the concept of covenant to characterize this relationship. Currently, however, nurses face a variety of obstacles to performing their responsibilities to the handicapped infant under this covenant, and Martin briefly explores how this situation could be changed.

The Nurse's Role

Responsibilities and Rights

Marsha D. M. Fowler

There is general agreement among nursing theorists that the root concepts of nursing are: nursing, health, person, and environment or society.[1] These concepts, together, comprise the metaparadigm of nursing and identify its distinctive scientific focus. In contrast, the metaparadigm concepts of medicine are: physician, pathophysiology, person, and society or environment. Every theory or model of nursing or of medicine will incorporate and define the profession's metaparadigm concepts and their linkages. Thus, although theories of medicine will differ among themselves, and theories of nursing will likewise differ, they will remain theories of medicine or nursing, by virtue of their incorporation of all of the particular root concepts of the profession.

Conceptually, nursing is defined as "the diagnosis and treatment of human responses to actual or potential health problems."[2] The phenomena of concern to nurses are, then, responses to health problems, rather than the problems or diseases that cause them. Thus, the focus of nursing *qua* nursing is rather different from the focus of medicine, though there are areas of overlapping concern. The definition, fundamental enterprise, concerns, ends, and goals of nursing differ from those of medicine. With difference comes a difference in the role, rights, responsibilities, and moral perspectives of nursing.

The Role of the Nurse

Contemporary nursing identifies itself as a "patient advocacy profession that includes a primary commitment to the patient. (In general, nursing identifies the "patient" as the individual with an actual or potential health problem plus that person's relational web. In some instances, the patient may be a group or a community, depending upon the nature of the nursing specialty.) Patient advocacy and a primary commitment to the patient are not new with nursing; this focus can be found in the earliest moral literature of the profession in this country.

As early as 1893, when Lystra Gretter wrote the Florence Nightingale Pledge, the first moral code for American nursing, one can see strands of commitment to the patient. The Pledge states "with loyalty will I aid the physician in his work and will devote myself to the welfare of those committed to my care."[3] The pledge does not state, as it has often been interpreted, that the nurse is devoted to the physician and loyal to the patient, and by implication that nursing is based upon an historical ethics of obedience. The object of nursing's concern and devotion was and remains the patient; nursing's ethics is rooted in a relationship with the patient and the well-being of that patient, not in an ethics of obedience. Where nursing has differed historically has been in its determination of how one goes about assuring the well-being of the patient. In earlier days it was often held that nursing best served the patient by adherence to the physician's orders. Contemporary nursing observes that the patient is best served by the independent (autonomous) practice of nursing as nursing, and collaborative practice with medicine where medical issues are of concern.

Both the Code for Nurses of the International Council of Nurses (ICN) and the American Nurses' Association (ANA) Code for Nurses support this position. The ICN code states that "The nurse's primary responsibility is to the people who require nursing care."[4] The ANA code declares that:

> The nurse's primary commitment is to the health, welfare, and safety of the client. As an advocate of the client, the nurse must be

alert to and take appropriate action regarding any instances of incompetent, unethical, or illegal practice by any member of the
health care team or the health care system, or any action on the part
of others that places the rights or best interests of the client in
jeopardy.[5]

The ANA Code additionally states that "professional autonomy
and self-regulation in the control of conditions of practice are necessary for implementing nursing standards."[6] In the ethics of the
profession today, nursing inextricably links advocacy for the patient with nursing autonomy and accountability as well.

Despite the fact that nursing so strongly aligns itself with the patient, in the role of advocate, the actual definition and development
of models of advocacy is as yet not well formulated. In general,
there are four emerging models of nursing advocacy; the specifica-
tion of the nurse's role and responsibilities within each model differs somewhat.

Models of Nursing Advocacy for the Patient: The Nurse's Responsibilities

One model, as propounded by Annas, Winslow, and others, proposes an essentially legal understanding of nursing advocacy as the
appropriate metaphor for nursing practice.[7] It "is associated with
virtues such as courage and norms such as the defense of the patient
against the infringement of his or her rights."[8] Those rights include
the patient's right to information about procedures, diagnosis, and
treatment; the right to accept or refuse medical intervention, the
right to leave the hospital, the right to be treated with respect, and
so forth.[9] In this form of advocacy, the nurse is responsible to be
well informed of the legal rights of the patient, and is willing to en-
ter into disputes to fight for those rights when they have been or will
be abridged.

This rights-based protection model of nursing advocacy is, in
part, supported by the Code for Nurses, which calls for the nurse to
act when "any action on the part of others...places the rights or best

interests of the patient in jeopardy."[10] Even so, the "best interests" clause muddies the waters somewhat, since the patient's best interests are not the focus of the rights-based model.[4] Despite Winslow's support of this model, Fry and others decry the use of a legal-rights conception of advocacy as the ideal for the nurse–patient relationship.[11,12]

Historically nursing has tended to consider itself to be based in an interpersonal, or perhaps even a moral, relationship to the patient rather than a legal one. Thus, a rights-protection model of advocacy strains at the boundaries of nursing's self identity and is much less comfortable a metaphor than one rooted in a more existential and less legal understanding of nursing's relationship with the patient.

Kohnke favors a values-based model of advocacy with a decisional counseling type of process of enactment. In this view of advocacy, the responsibility of the nurse is to seek to assist the patient in identifying or clarifying his or her own values, and to make a decision that is most congruent with, and the best expression of, those values.[13] Steps in this process would include supporting the patient and assisting the patient to clarify values, appraise the situation, survey and evaluate alternatives, and act upon (and adhere to) that position even in the face of negative feedback.[14,15]

Gadow espouses a variant form of this view of advocacy. She sees advocacy as "existential advocacy," and proposes that:

> The philosophical foundation and ideal of nursing is that of advocacy—not the concept of advocacy implied in the patients' rights movement, in which any health professional potentially is a consumer advocate, but a fundamental, existential advocacy for which the nurse alone, among all the health professionals, is uniquely suited, and which is as distinct from consumer advocacy as it is from paternalism.[16]

For Gadow, the role of the nurse in existential advocacy does not "consist in protecting the individuals' rights to do what they want," but rather:

> To help persons become clear about what they want to do, by helping them discern and clarify their values in the situation, and on the basis of that self-examination, to reach decisions which ex-

press their reaffirmed, perhaps recreated (by the illness), complex of values.[17]

Unfortunately, the values-based decisional model of nursing advocacy requires a patient who is self-determining (as an expression of values), or whose values could be known either through the family or through an instrument such as the durable power of attorney for health care. Thus, it is not sufficient as a model to encompass the patient who cannot participate in the decisional process or whose values can not be known.

Such a patient makes a third model of advocacy necessary. Fry has referred to this model as the "respect-for-persons" model and cites Murphy's perspective on this model.[18] Murphy has referred to the respect-for-persons model as the "patient-advocate model," a designation that is now insufficiently descriptive. This model demands that the nurse respect the dignity and personhood of the patient whether or not the patient is self-determining or autonomous. When the patient is self-determining (or has a surrogate decision maker), the nurse functions in a fashion similar to the values-based decisional model. However, when the patient is non-autonomous, and there is no one to speak for the patient, the nurse is called to act in the "best interests" of the patient, as defined by the nurse. Murphy maintains that the nurse is in the best position to make these judgments, largely owing to the amount of time the nurse spends with the individual patient, and the continuous, caring nature of the nurse–patient relationship.[19]

It is ultimately this model of advocacy that the Code for Nurses supports, despite its mention of protection of patient rights. This model demands that the nurse advocate be accountable directly to the patient for having served in his or her best interests, and accountable to society for the judgments made as an advocate for either the autonomous or nonautonomous patient.

Not all advocacy, however, takes place at the bedside. A "larger," more political perspective on nursing advocacy forms a fourth model. It is best typified by Freeman's notion of "practice as protest," which contains an element of bedside advocacy, but extends to social advocacy as a form of social criticism and social change. Freeman envisions three major ways in which nurses can practice/ protest:

1. We can engage in public contest and confrontation, sharing the cause of the aggrieved.
2. We can act as advocates for those we serve, fighting the battles little and big—that they are ill prepared to fight for themselves.
3. We can, through the practice of nursing itself, build the capability of those we serve so they are able to fend for themselves, to earn their own place in the sun or fight for rights withheld.[20]

For Freeman, this form of advocacy does more than secure care for an individual. It is a means of calling to the attention of providers of care the inconsistencies and inadequacies of care.[21] It is rooted in a concept of social justice and is an attempt to get at and correct system-wide inequities and injustices that lead to care that fails to respect the rights, values, or dignity of the patient.

None of the four models above has been fully developed; they are emerging models of advocacy that have yet to be articulated in theory and tested in practice. Elements of each of these models can be seen throughout the nursing literature, and it remains to be seen which will emerge as the model with the greatest explanatory power in the light of the ethical norms and tradition of the profession.

The Nurse's Rights as Patient Advocate

The Right to Protection from Reprisal

In a recent statement of the ANA Committee on Ethics, entitled "Ethics of Safeguarding Client Health and Safety," elements of each of the models of advocacy are evident, though there is a very strong emphasis on collective nursing action for social change. Collective action is not, however, merely for the purposes of bringing about social change through the power of a unified voice. Collective action also serves to protect individual nurses from possible retaliation for acting upon the moral norms of the profession.

The issue of the protection of the nurse who questions the moral or legal or medical appropriateness of another's actions has been a consistent concern within the profession. As the Code notes,

> There should be an established process for the reporting and handling of incompetent, unethical, or illegal practice within the employment setting so that such reporting can go through official channels without fear of reprisal.[22]

So too, the Committee notes that "collective action by the nursing profession is required in order to minimize the individual heroism and risk-taking often required in 'whistle-blowing' situations."[23] If the advocacy role of the nurse generates responsibilities toward or on behalf of the patient, and both the profession and the institution demand fulfillment of those responsibilities, the nurse has a right to act in accord with those duties without fear of reprisal.

The Nurse's Right to Institutional Processes and Procedures

Advocacy as a contemporary metaphor for nursing practice is sufficiently large to encompass other role obligations addressed by the Code for Nurses and the ethical literature of the profession. Such responsibilities include duties of acting nonprejudicially toward patients, maintaining confidentiality, respecting privacy, assuming accountability and responsibility for nursing judgments, maintaining competence, refusing an inappropriate assignment, developing the profession's body of knowledge, maintaining and improving the standards of the profession, assuring working conditions conducive to high-quality nursing care, maintaining the integrity of the profession, and collaborating with other health professionals to meet the health needs of the public.

In all this, however, the nurse cannot act upon the moral obligations the profession propounds without having adequate safeguards, as noted above, and viable processes or mechanisms in place. Herein lie, at least in part, the nurse's rights correlative to responsibilities. If a nurse is enjoined to act upon moral judgments, that nurse has a right to expect established processes for such action. The Code states that:

> to function effectively in this role [as patient advocate] nurses
> must be aware of the employing institution's policies and proce-
> dures, nursing standards of practice, the Code for Nurses, and laws
> governing nursing and health care practice with regard to incompe-
> tent, unethical, or illegal practice.[24]

As an aside, it is clear that in order to judge the appropriateness
of the actions of others (whether physician, nurse, or family member) relative to the patient's best interests, nurses must have extensive knowledge of professional codes and standards, laws that govern nursing and health care practice, and medical therapeutics.
Note that although the law may declare a nurse not legally qualified
to judge medical competence, the ethics of the profession nonetheless requires it.

The nurse's judgments are to be made over against these and
other standards. Action based upon such judgments is dependent
upon the existence of institutional processes. Generally, either or
both of two major avenues of pursuit are available.

The Traditional Route of Patient Advocacy

The first route of patient advocacy is the traditional, upward,
hierarchical reporting within the institution, with resort to noninsti-
tutional authorities within the health care system when the various
levels of the hierarchy are refractory to expressions of concern.
This particular process involves immediate communication with
the person judged not to be acting in the patient's best interests, factual documentation, memoranda of concern, and other written
instruments as directed by the institution's policies. These rise to
succeeding levels within the hierarchy, until such time as the situation is resolved.

A process of this nature is generally cumbersome, laborious,
subject to interruption or delay, and often ineffectual. It is, however, accessible to all nurses. Every nurse has a right to expect that
an institution will have formalized policies and procedures for
reporting illegal, incompetent, or morally inappropriate behavior,

and perhaps a different mechanism for each kind of problem. The nurse has both a right and responsibility to utilize the mechanisms in place, and to use them without penalty, before going outside established lines of communication.

Emerging Routes

A second and increasingly more efficient and effective avenue for patient advocacy is the institutional ethics committee (IEC), which is meant to address issues or problems of an ethical nature. (Questions of competence are often better addressed by peer review or quality assessment committees. Questions of lawfulness should be directed to other groups, depending upon the nature and context of the presumed illegal practice. In some instances, illegal practice should be reported to licensing boards; in others to the district attorney or other legal bodies.)

In 1984, the House of Delegates of the ANA adopted a resolution that encouraged state nurses' associations to:

> promote nurses' active participation in the development, implementation, and evaluation of formal mechanisms for multidisciplinary institutional ethical review such as institutional ethics committees.[25]

The ANA Committee on Ethics subsequently prepared guidelines to assist nurses in establishing and participating in the work of an IEC. The Committee noted that:

> The impetus for the development of such mechanisms arises out of ethical, legal, and social concerns that include an increasing dissatisfaction on the part of both health care professionals and consumers with existing institutional decision-making processes, and the difficult moral choices that directly and indirectly affect patient/client care and welfare.[26]

Nursing's concern for the development of IECs is specifically to protect the quality of patient care and the welfare, well-being, and interests of the patient.

Although in the stage of clinical trial, the IEC is proving a useful mechanism for the resolution or prevention of moral dilemmas that affect the quality of patient care. IECs are perhaps most effective in quasi-legislative, rather than quasi-judicial, functions. Some categories of moral dilemmas in nursing practice, which jeopardize either the rights or best interests of the patient, are recurrent. When nurses raise these issues to an IEC, that group can prepare general guidelines for efficiently and effectively handling a specific category of problem. When nurses remain silent, guidelines may never be developed.

Although the nurse has the right to expect that institutions will have procedures for reporting illegal, incompetent, or unethical behavior, and mechanisms (such as IECs) for their resolution, the nurse also has a duty to utilize the procedures that do exist and to assist in their development when they do not. That is, the nurse is expected to actively participate in establishing the work environment, moral milieu, or procedures wherein the right of nurses to practice as patient advocates can be realized.

"Patient advocacy" is clearly the watchword of this era of nursing. It is not, of course, an end in itself, but rather a means to effect the nurturative, generative, and supportive practices of nursing, which focus the profession's attention on "health"; for health is "the center of nursing attention, not as an end in itself, but as a means to life that is meaningful and manageable."[27] The nurse is responsible to the patient and to society insofar as she or he has worked toward achieving that end.

Notes And References

[1] Jacqueline Fawcett (1984) *Analysis and Evaluation of Conceptual Models of Nursing* F. A. Davis, Philadelphia.

[2] American Nurses' Association (1980) *Nursing: A Social Policy Statement* American Nurses' Association, Kansas City, MO.

[3] Lystra Gretter (1893) *The Florence Nightingale Pledge* Lystra Gretter.

[4] International Council of Nurses (1973) *Code For Nurses* Geneva, ICN.

[5] American Nurses' Association (1985) *Code for Nurses with Interpretive Statements,* Kansas City, MO, ANA.

[6]Ibid.

[7]Winslow, G. (1984) From Loyalty to Advocacy: A New Metaphor for Nursing, *Hastings Center Report* **14**(3), pp. 32–40.

[8]Ibid., p. 32.

[9]Ibid., p. 36.

[10]Code p. 6.

[11]Fry, S. T. (1984) Ethics in Community Health Nursing Practice, in *Community Health Nursing* (L. Lancaster and M. Stanhope, eds.) St. Louis, MO, Mosby, pp. 77–96.

[12]Fowler, M. D. M. (1984) *Ethics in Nursing, 1893–1984: The Ideal of Service, The Reality of History* Los Angeles, University of Southern California.

[13]Kohnke, M. E. (1980) The Nurse as Advocate. *American Journal of Nursing,* **80**: 2038–2040.

[14]Uustal, D. (1987) Values: Cornerstone of Nurses' Moral Art, in *Ethics at the Bedside* (M. Fowler and J. Levine–Ariff, eds.) Philadelphia, Lippincott, pp. 136–170

[15]Janis, I. (1983) *Short-Term Counseling.* New Haven, Yale University Press, p. 137.

[16]Spicker, S. and Gadow, S. (1980) *Nursing Images and Ideals: Opening Dialogue with the Humanities* New York, Springer, p. 81.

[17]Ibid., p. 85.

[18]Fry, S. T. (1987) Autonomy, Advocacy, and Accountability: Ethics at the Bedside, *Ethics at the Bedside* (M. Fowler and J. Levine–Ariff, eds.) Philadelphia, Lippincott, pp. 39–50. I am indebted to Dr. Fry for her typology of models of advocacy.

[19]Murphy, C. P. (1983) Models of the Nurse-Patient Relationship, in *Ethical Problems in the Nurse–Patient Relationship* (C. P. Murphy and H. Hunter, eds.) Boston, Allyn and Bacon, pp. 9–24.

[20]Freeman, R. (1971) Practice as Protest. *American Journal of Nursing* **71**: 5, 918–921.

[21]Ibid., p. 920.

[22]Code, p. 6.

[23]Committee on Ethics, American Nurses' Association (December 1986) *Ethics of Safeguarding Client Health and Safety,* Kansas City, MO, ANA.

[24]Code, p. 6

[25]American Nurses' Association (1986) *Guidelines for Nurses' Participation and Leadership in Institutional Ethical Review Processes,* Kansas City, MO, ANA.

[26]Ibid.

[27]ANA, Social Policy Statement, p. 6.

The Legacy of Baby Doe

Nurses' Ethical and Legal Obligations
to Severely Handicapped Newborns

Darlene Aulds Martin

Introduction

"Baby Doe" has become imbedded in our public consciousness, a visible symbol of the controversy surrounding the withholding of treatment from newborns with serious handicaps. The infant behind the name was born with symptoms of Down's syndrome and tracheoesophageal fistula (an abnormal connection between the trachea and esophagus) in April, 1982 in Bloomington, Indiana. Although the fistula was surgically correctable, the parents made the decision to forego surgery based on advice from their obstetrician that chances for successful repair of the fistula were limited and that the infant would be seriously retarded. The parents' decision to withhold surgery as well as feedings and hydration was legally challenged, but sustained in both the trial and appeals court in Indiana. Left untreated, Baby Doe died on the sixth day of life before a court-appointed attorney could obtain review in the US Supreme Court.[1]

The case dramatically thrust the issue of non-treatment into the public arena and generated an intense national debate concerning the constitutional rights of handicapped newborns, the boundaries

157

of parental decision-making, the ethical-legal obligations of medical professionals toward infants and parents, and the legitimacy of governmental intervention in treatment decisions. The ensuing debate precipitated a series of legislative, judicial, and regulatory responses at both state and federal levels. These responses culminated in the recent enactment of amendments to the Federal Child Abuse Prevention and Treatment Act of 1974.[2]

Although it is too soon to gauge the full impact of the new regulations, it is apparent that this attempted remedy has not stilled the debate over treatment of handicapped newborns. The regulations are a compromise measure forged by a fragile alliance of medical, child advocacy, pro-life, and political groups who were each seeking to advance their own perspective about treatment. The continuing controversy underscores the fact that there remains a climate of mistrust and profound philosophical differences among these groups that are not easily reconciled. Many of the child advocates believe that regulations are absolutely necessary to protect the civil rights of handicapped infants, whereas many in the medical community believe that the regulations are an unwarranted intrusion into clinical practice.

It is clear that a just and humane resolution of these complex treatment dilemmas will require a collective engagement of all parties in honest and substantive dialog. These dilemmas do not lend themselves to quick fixes or simple, reductionist formulas, but rather call out for reasoned, compassionate approaches that focus on the best interest of the child.

Regrettably, much of the dialog concerning the treatment dilemma has failed to incorporate the special perspective of neonatal intensive care nurses. Yet these nurses are thrust into the "eye of the storm" as the primary caregivers who support and sustain these infant patients during this critical time in their lives. From the beginning, there is an intimate connection that inextricably binds the nurse and infant. In many ways, the nurse becomes part of the baby's ecosystem—assessing, restoring, nurturing, comforting, and sometimes, accompanying unto death. It is a powerful role that fuses healer and parent-surrogate into one and transcends the perception of nurses as "high-tech" engineers. I will advance the claim that this unique relationship creates an ethical warrant and a *prima facie* duty for the nurse to advocate for treatment that is in the best interest of the infant. The saliency of this claim has been underscored by the pivotal role of neonatal nurses in the "Baby Doe" case and other significant legal cases involving nontreatment of handicapped newborns.

This paper will explore the nature of the nurse's ethical-legal obligations to these vulnerable infants in light of current regulations and litigation. To provide a framework for examining these obligations, I will briefly trace the evolution of the treatment dilemma and outline substantive ethical-legal issues that are inherent in the dilemma.

Historical Development of Treatment Dilemmas

Historically, the dilemma of treatment for severely handicapped newborns is not a new issue. Infants and children with handicaps have always been part of our reality, and our society has often struggled with the issue of their care. What is new, however, is the growing magnitude and complexity of the treatment dilemma, as well as the degree to which it has come under public scrutiny. In many respects, the dilemma is a by-product of the technological revolution in medicine. Rapidly advancing medical technology has provided the means for treating and sustaining many premature and severely handicapped infants who would have died a decade ago. Approximately four percent of the annual 3.3 million live births in the US are infants who have multiple congenital anomalies. An additional seven percent of live births, or 230,000 infants, weigh 2500 grams or less at birth and sustain high risks for developing significant anomalies as well as premature death.[3]

Although it is clear that many of these infants have benefited substantially from new and aggressive medical therapies, there are troubling questions about the humaneness of aggressive treatment for certain infants such as those who are severely premature, irreversibly dying, or for whom treatment outcomes may be unknown or deleterious, as well as for certain infants with severe, permanent mental and physiological impairments. These questions are intrinsically tied to a larger societal inquiry into the appropriate uses and limits of life-saving technology. A decade of prolonged debate punctuated by the cases of Karen Ann Quinlan[4], Brother Fox[5], and Elizabeth Bouvia[6] has focused unprecedented attention on ethical and legal issues surrounding the care of terminally ill and/or irreversibly comatose patients.

Although public sentiment and judicial opinions have generally tended to support the decisions of competent, adult patients and families of incompetent adults to forego life-sustaining treatment, there remains sharp controversy about withholding such treatment from severely handicapped newborns. At the heart of the dilemma are conflicting beliefs about whether it is ever morally and legally justifiable to allow multi-handicapped infants to die by withholding treatment or food. In more graphic terms, as posed by Lyon, should the withholding of treatment be considered a benevolent act of compassion or is it an act of murder?[7]

Conflicting Beliefs About Withholding Treatment

Attempts to justify or refute withholding life-sustaining treatment have often turned on vastly different concepts of the infant as person. Several commentators have argued that withholding treatment from severely handicapped infants can be justified on the grounds that they do not meet the specific criteria for or have the requisite characteristics of "personhood." Fletcher's notion of personhood is reflected in his "humanhood profile," a description of characteristics that he believes entitles one to be called "person."

These include minimal intelligence, self-awareness, a sense of past and future time, and the capability of relating to others.[8] Tooley advances the argument that "personhood" and the right to life are based on an organism's development of the concept of a continuing self. He believes that mental impairment of many handicapped infants would preclude their evolving such a knowledge of self.[9]

These arguments denying the "humanhood" of severely handicapped infants seem to be an attempt to define the infants out of existence rather than to confront the hard questions about the nature of care that is the most humane. From an ethical view, I would argue that these infants share an inherent "humanness" with all of us, irrespective of their probable mentality or awareness of self, and that common bond should guide decisions made on their behalf. From a legal perspective, it is clear that infants are considered persons who are protected by full constitutional rights.[10]

Others have asserted that withholding treatment is justified since in their view many handicapped infants, especially those with severe mental impairment, will not be able to develop meaningful human relationships or engage in other activities that give life purpose. McCormick articulated this position in an early paper, "To Save or Let Die," in which he made the claim that "life is a relative good and the duty to preserve it a limited one."[11]

At the other end of the spectrum are those who hold that life-sustaining treatment should always be given irrespective of the severity of the handicaps because of traditional societal commitments to the principles of sanctity of life and respect for persons. Ramsey calls into question the measurement of an infant's life based solely on potential. He states, "Persons are not reducible to their potential, we need only ask what fidelity to another human life, perhaps lacking any further potential and lacking reciprocity, requires of an (moral) agent."[12] Other advocates for mandatory treatment of severely handicapped newborns believe that many of these infants, with assistance, can develop meaningful lives and can, indeed, contribute to society. These advocates believe that many handicapped newborns are subjected to nontreatment decisions based on either blatant discrimination, especially if there is a risk of mental retardation, or lack of accurate information about handicapping conditions.[13,14] Koop, the current US Surgeon General, argues that physicians who withhold treatment from non-dying handicapped newborns are, in effect, condoning infanticide. He believes that their actions are often based on attempts to prevent parents from being burdened.[15]

Best Interest Standard

While respecting the claim that all infants have inherent worth and are deserving of medical care, I would also support the claim that under certain very restricted conditions an infant may be better and more lovingly served by foregoing very aggressive medical therapy. This position, referred to as the "best interest" standard, holds that it may be morally justifiable to withhold life-sustaining treatment from certain infants if it can be determined that treatment is not in their best interest.[16]

This view attempts to ground decision-making more solidly on the *child's* best interest rather than to focus on the interests of other parties or to relegate the infant to the land of non-persons. Fost has argued the need for a best interest standard:

"Neither a pro-life policy of treating all infants maximally, or a permissive policy of allowing all parents to decide can be defended. The former position leads to the *reductio ad absurdum* of trying to keep everyone alive forever. The latter gives rise to empiric abuses such as starvation of infants with good prospects for happiness and self-sufficiency, as well as the conceptual difficulty of claiming that parental authority over children includes the right to engineer their death if the child's existence threatens parental happiness.[17]"

Although the notion of decision-making based on "best interest" has a strong intuitive appeal, it has several inherent difficulties that need to be addressed. First, there is a lack of substantive criteria that could be used as the basis for decision-making, and second, a lack of well-established processes or procedures for decision-making that would in fact be protective of the child's best interests. The attempt to develop criteria for treatment is complicated by the significant amount of diagnostic and prognostic uncertainty that may accompany many severe handicapping conditions. It may be difficult to predict a seriously ill infant's chances of surviving multiple surgeries or experimental treatments, the degree of future physical and/or mental impairment, or the degree of chronic pain. Many of the hardest cases fall into what Fost has characterized as "... the vast and ill-defined gray zone."[18]

Bartholome has used the metaphor of a "conceptual swamp" to describe the inherent perplexity and ambiguity that attends decision-making in the NICU. He believes that the best interest standard, although not a substantive criterion, can serve as a light or beacon to guide decision-makers.[19] Bartholome has proposed that one means of trying to determine whether treatment is in the child's best interest would be to plot the "trajectory" of the infant's response to treatment over time. If it can be established that the infant is clearly not responding to treatment, that his or her condition is actually deteriorating, or that he or she is becoming substantially *more* dependent on technology, e.g., mechanical respirator, to survive, then there may be justification for foregoing life-sustaining treatment.[20]

Weir has proposed the concept of "selective nontreatment" of infants with certain handicaps utilizing criteria that are based on diagnostic categories. Decisions to treat are characterized as either obligatory or optional, depending on the relative benefits and harms to the infant from the proposed treatment modalities. [21]

Although there appears to be some consensus among those who advocate the use of the best interest standard about withholding treatment from infants who are excessively premature or who are irreversibly dying or comatose, there is substantial disagreement about foregoing treatment of conditions such as spina bifida cystica, which may result in varying degrees of permanent physical and mental impairments. Unfortunately, the lack of consensus has frequently led to inconsistent, and at times, inequitable treatment decisions for handicapped newborns.

A striking example of that disagreement is reflected in the vastly different medical approaches to spina bifida. Lorber has advocated the use of specific clinical criteria as the basis for making treatment decisions for children with spina bifida in England. Those infants with severe spina bifida who are judged according to Lorber's criteria to have a poor prognostic course are not treated aggressively and usually die within several months.[22] Although Lorber's criteria have been adopted by physicians in a number of countries, many physicians in the US, including Freeman[23], McClone[24], and Shurtleff[25] have challenged the reliability of Lorber's clinical criteria. They have also pointed out the significant problems that occur when infants with spina bifida are left untreated but manage to survive. They advocate aggressive treatment for the majority of infants with spina bifida because of research that indicates good surgical and medical outcomes for many of the infants.

The intensity of the debate over selective treatment of children with spina bifida was recently dramatized by a lawsuit filed against the Oklahoma Children's Memorial Hospital seeking to halt their use of "quality of life" criteria as the basis for decision-making. The suit alleged that 24 infants with myelogeningocele died because they were denied medically beneficial treatment during the course of an experimental study at the hospital. The Federal court in *Johnson v Gross* decided that the infants' constitutional rights had been violated.[26]

In addition to a lack of concensus about the criteria for decision-making, there is controversy about both the process that should be utilized as well as the persons who should be involved in making decisions on behalf of handicapped newborns. In general, there is a presupposition in the law that parents should have the right to make decisions on behalf of their minor children as long as those decisions are in keeping with the child's best interest. That right, however, is not absolute. Parents bear a legal duty to provide necessary medical care for their children, and the state may intercede if the child's life or health is seriously threatened.[27-31]

Robertson has argued that the stress that surrounds the birth of a handicapped infant may be so great that it may preclude the parents' ability to make objective treatment decisions. He believes that nontreat decisions should be reviewed by ethics committees and, if necessary, by courts in order to assure that just decision-making has occurred.[32]

Private Decision-Making Goes Public

The practice of withholding treatment as well as the process of making treatment decisions has come under intense professional and public scrutiny only during the past decade. Prior to that time, decisions for initiating or withholding treatment were made by the physician and parents with little public attention or concern. These decisions were viewed, generally, as private matters between the physician and parents, with the physician relying on his or her judgment, as well as the preferences of the parents.

The essentially private practice of withholding treatment from certain handicapped newborns was brought sharply into public view through a series of cases reported in the early 1970s. The first of these was a compelling case at Johns Hopkins Hospital involving an infant with Down's syndrome and duodenal atresia whose parents made the decision not to have the atresia surgically corrected because they did not want to raise a child who was mentally retarded. The attending physician concurred with their decision. Without repair of the duodenal defect, the infant was unable to receive oral feedings and died 15 days later.

This case stimulated a series of articles in professional journals[33,34] as well as the production of a film, "Who Shall Survive," depicting the events that occurred in the Johns Hopkins case.[35] The film was produced by the Joseph P. Kennedy, Jr. Foundation in Washington, DC, and raised crucial questions about the basis for decision making, especially in cases involving neonates with mental retardation. The rights of parents to be final decision makers and the obligations of physicians and nurses to both infants and parents were also examined.

The extent of the practice of withholding treatment from handicapped neonates was further emphasized in a study by Duff and Campbell[36] who reported 43 cases of passive euthanasia in the newborn nursery at the Yale-New Haven Hospital during 1973. They noted that these cases involved deliberate decisions by physicians and/or parents not to treat this group of handicapped newborns. The widespread use of passive euthanasia as a treatment of choice with selected infants was further underscored by physicians' testimony to a select Senate subcommittee convened to examine ethical issues in medicine.[37] In addition, a number of surveys of pediatricians and pediatric surgeons reported that these medical professionals had participated in, or would consider using such practices in, a wide range of cases involving handicapped neonates.[38-40]

More recently, public attention focused on the issue of non-treatment in three highly publicized cases in Illinois, Indiana, and New York. The Danville, Illinois case involved Siamese twins who were born joined together at the waist and shared three legs. The attending obstetrician and the father of the infants, also a physician, concurred in a decision not to treat the infants immediately after delivery, and a "no feed" order was noted in the medical record. Several nurses in the neonatal unit complained to the physician about the lack of feeding, and on several occasions the infants were fed by one or more of the nurses. One week after the birth, an anonymous phone call alerted the Illinois Department of Children and Family Services that the infants were being denied care. After an investigation, the Child and Family Services Department was awarded temporary custody of the infants, and they were taken to a Chicago hospital for a series of medical evaluations and treatments. At one year of age, the twins were surgically separated.

The case is unique in that the District Attorney attempted to prosecute the physicians and parents in a criminal action for conspiracy to commit murder. At a preliminary hearing to establish probable cause, however, no witnesses could link any of the parties to the actual signing of the order not to feed and the case was dismissed. The court has since issued a ruling that the children could be returned to the custody of their parents.[41]

Baby Doe Regulations

The Indiana case, discussed earlier as "Baby Doe," generated a massive public response as well as a personal one from President Reagan. In May, 1982, President Reagan instructed the Secretary of Health and Human Services (HHS) to issue a directive to hospitals across the country informing them of the potential loss of federal funds if they withheld nutritional sustenance or medical or surgical treatment from handicapped infants. The authority for the threatened withholding was the Reagan administration's interpretation of Section 504 of the Rehabilitation Act of 1973, which forbids a recipient of Federal financial assistance from denying an individual the benefits of a program solely on the basis of handicap.[42]

In March, 1983, HHS proposed a formal regulation specifying that hospitals that received Federal financial assistance must display a poster that detailed the illegality of denying customary medical care or nutrition to handicapped infants.[43] In addition, the poster carried the requirement that any person who was aware of violations of the regulation should contact a newly established National Handicapped Infant Hotline, which would trigger an on-site investigation. The regulation further provided that HHS would have authority to act to protect a reported infant. The regulation was intended to take effect immediately, ignoring the required minimum 30-day notice and comment period specified in the Federal Administrative Procedures Act.[44]

Negative response from much of the medical community resulted in a suit being filed against HHS by the American Academy of Pediatrics, the National Association of Children's Hospitals, and the Children's Hospital National Medical Center. On April 14, 1983, US District Judge Gerhard Gesell issued a ruling that the regulation was illegal because of HHS's failure to follow proper procedures in putting forth the regulation. Judge Gesell further commented on the potentially disruptive effects that could occur with the use of Baby Doe hotlines and investigative teams.[45] The Department of Health and Human Services revised the regulations and resubmitted them for public comment. These regulations were later struck down in a series of judicial opinions discussed below.

Baby Jane Doe

Following closely behind the case of Baby Doe was a third and perhaps more graphically publicized case involving a baby girl who came to be known as "Baby Jane Doe." Born on October 11, 1983, on Long Island, New York, Baby Jane sustained multiple congenital handicaps, including myelomeningocele at L-3 to L-4, hydrocephalus, and microcephaly. In addition, she had spasticity in her upper extremities and a prolapsed rectum.

Initial medical evaluations indicated that the infant would probably have significant paralysis of her lower limbs and severe mental retardation. After consultation with physicians, clergy, and family members, the parents requested that physicians forego surgical repair of the baby's myelomeningocele and proceed with a conservtive course of medical intervention including antibiotics and nutritional support. The infant's physicians at Stonybrook concurred with the parents' decision and initiated a medical regimen. However, within a few days, an anonymous member of the hospital staff alerted Lawrence Washburn, an attorney who was very involved in the right to life movement in a neighboring state. Washburn initiated legal action to force surgical treatment of the infant.[46]

Following an evidentiary hearing of the case, Justice Melvyn Tanenbaum ruled that the infant must have corrective surgery. The parents' attorney filed an immediate appeal, and one day later an appellate panel of the New York Supreme Court reversed the earlier ruling and allowed a course of conservative therapy to be initiated. The court stated that "concerned and loving parents have made an informed, intelligent, and reasonable determination based upon and supported by responsible medical authority."[47] The New York Court of Appeals upheld the decision by the Appellate court on the grounds that Mr. Washburn did not have standing to bring the suit and that he had not appropriately contacted state welfare authorities to initiate action.[48]

During the ensuing legal action, the Federal government also became involved via a Justice Department suit requesting that Stonybrook Hospital turn over Baby Jane Doe's medical records. Access was denied by both the US Court of Appeals, which raised questions whether, under Section 504, the neonatal unit was a "recipient" of Federal financial assistance; whether corrective surgery was a "program" and whether there was discrimination, i.e. would the surgery have been performed if the infant were not handicapped?[49] The US Supreme Court, in *Bowen* v *American Hospital Association*, affirmed the lower court's denial of governmental access to records and invalidated the basis upon which the Reagan Administration had promulgated the "Baby Doe" regulations.[50]

Although there has been some misperception that the Supreme Court ruling struck down the only law governing decision-making about newborns, the new child abuse amendments shift responsibility of protecting handicapped infants to the states.

It is interesting to note that in the midst of the litigation and regulation, the parents of Baby Jane made a decision to allow physicians to establish a shunt to decrease the baby's hydrocephaly. Following surgery, Baby Jane was taken home by her parents.

Child Abuse Amendments

Following in the wake of the Baby Jane Doe controversy, there was increased activity by some members of Congress in pushing for further handicapped infant protections. In the summer of 1984, the US House and Senate drafted legislation that incorporated the withholding of medically indicated treatment from handicapped infants into the existing Federal Child Abuse Prevention and Treatment Act of 1974. The legislation mandated that child protective agencies in each state monitor the treatment of handicapped newborns and initiate legal action when necessary. The proposed legislation was signed into law as PL 98-457 by President Reagan on October 9, 1984[52] and accompanying regulations promulgated in 1985.[53]

Although the legislation specifies that medical treatment that would ameliorate or correct a life-threatening condition must be given, it provides that such treatment may be withheld under the following circumstances:

(1) the infant is chronically and irreversibly comatose,

(2) the treatment will merely prolong dying,

(3) the treatment would be futile in terms of the infant's survival and the treatment "itself under such circumstances would by inhumane."[54]

An additional important feature of this law is the emphasis on the establishment of Infant Care Review Committees within hospitals, particularly those with tertiary level neonatal care units. The purpose of the Infant Care Committees is to establish guidelines and policies regarding the withholding of treatment of handicapped newborns, as well as to provide counsel and review of cases in which withholding of treatment is being considered. The Department of Health and Human Services has published model ICRC guidelines describing the composition of the committee (which should include a practicing professional nurse), as well as the role of the committee in developing policy, reviewing cases, and serving as an educational resource for staff and families of handicapped infants.

During this time of debate, the issue of treatment for seriously handicapped newborns was also addressed by the President's Commission for the Study of Ethical Principles in Medicine and Biomedical and Behavioral Research in their report "Deciding to Forego Life-Sustaining Treatment."[55] The Commission emphasized the need for hospitals to establish specific policies that would govern decision making with seriously ill newborns. An important component of these policies would be a mechanism for internal review of decisions, especially in cases where therapy would not be undertaken or would be discontinued or in which there is a disagreement among medical professionals and parents/surrogates as to the treat/no treat decision. The Commission felt that internal review policies were preferable to governmental regulations.

In evaluating the circumstances under which an infant with permanent handicaps would be treated, the Commission concluded that "a very restrictive standard is appropriate: such permanent handicaps justify a decision not to provide life-sustaining treatment only when they are so severe that continued existence would not be a net benefit to the infant."[56]

Although the full weight of the new regulations and judicial opinions upon treatment decisions cannot yet be accurately evaluated, it may be substantial. There will undoubtedly be closer scrutiny of all nontreatment decisions by child protective agencies and others to determine if withholding treatment meets new Federal definitions of child abuse. If child abuse, as defined by the regulations, is found to exist, parents, physicians, nurses, and others who participated in nontreatment decisions and/or implementation of those decisions may be subject to prosecution.

Nurses' Ethical-Legal Obligations to Infants

In the face of the continuing controversy and evolving litigation and regulations, I believe that it is crucial for nurses to redefine the nature and scope of their commitments to infant patients and to assert their legitimate claims as participants in the decision-making process regarding treatment of severely handicapped newborns.

Although neonatal nurses as a group have always been vitally concerned about the welfare of their infant patients, they have often been unsure about the exact nature and extent of their ethical-legal obligations in securing that welfare. The uncertainty may stem, in part, from a sense of conflicting loyalties and competing claims that derive from nurses' "multiple ethical obligations."[57] Nurses frequently feel that they are caught in a cross-fire between legitimate duties owed to the institution, the primary physician, the infant's parents, and their infant patient. Whose claim has primacy?

Traversing the maze of conflicting obligations requires nurses to change their "conceptual roadmaps"—to refocus on the commitments that flow from the nurse-infant relationship. It is especially important for nurses and others who work with infants and children to understand that their *primary* obligations are to the infant patient. This is a crucial issue in neonatology and pediatrics because clinicians may lose sight of "who" the patient is as they interact closely with parents and others on the infant's behalf. The interests of the infant may recede into the background as parents and other health professionals voice their own claims. The Nurses' Professional Code of Ethics makes it clear, however, that the patient is the primary focus of concern.[58] This is not to negate the obligations that nurses have to parents and other health professionals who care for the infant, but to suggest that those claims and interests have to be weighed and balanced against those of the infant.

Nurses as Existential Advocates

I made an earlier claim that the nurse's significant care giving role with its intimate and extended view of the infant creates a strong advocacy obligation. It is not a claim borne out of territorial rights, but rather an acknowledgment of the unique healer/surrogate-mother role of the nurse. The advocacy obligation presupposes that the nurse enters into a covenantal or fiduciary relationship with the infant that will hold fast through time and circumstance. The covenant is irrevocable —it is not abandoned at the change of shifts or in the face of adversity. I believe that establishing such covenantal relationships is a moral requirement for professional nurses as an explicit symbol of their enduring and binding commitments.

Gadow has argued that the philosophical core of nursing practice should be grounded in an ethic of existential advocacy. This conception of advocacy would cast nurses in the role of facilitators — assisting patients to explore the meaning of their illness according to their own values and to "authentically exercise their freedom of self-determination" in making decisions about their care.[59] It is a complex and demanding notion that would require nurses to become more engaged in the process of preserving patient autonomy.

Although this model of advocacy has been primarily discussed by Gadow in relation to the care of adults, it seems, intuitively, to fit the role of nurses in the neonatal intensive care unit. Of all the health professionals who care for the infant during his or her neonatal stay, the nurses probably have the most intense and enduring contact. Collectively, they provide comprehensive, a-round-the-clock care to the infant, constantly assessing and ministering to his or her needs. From that intensive, close-up view, primary care nurses become experts at reading and interpreting the infant's physiological and psychological responses to the myriad of treatments, diagnostic procedures, and surgeries that he or she may undergo. Over time, they develop an encyclopedic knowledge of the infant's problems and successes and often note small, subtle changes that may be missed by others, such as a difference in cry or increased eye movements. They may be the first to recognize significant shifts in the infant's overall status, e.g., crossing over the line from critically ill to dying or rallying from coma to conscious-ness.

In some respects, the nurses become the infant's life-line, an attachment to the world around him or her. Because of this close connection, they are in a unique position to serve as advocates, to help give voice to the nature of the infant's experience, and to help shape decisions that are in the infant's best interest. In the face of decisions that they deem to not be in the infant's best interest, nurses bear both an ethical and a legal obligation to take action.

The ethical responsibility to act on the infant's behalf derives from the covenant between nurse and infant and a professional ethic grounded in the principles of beneficence, fidelity, veracity, and justice. Legal responsibility to act in the face of possible harm to the infant derives from the nurses' independent legal liability for their own actions and comparative liability relative to the actions of others. Nurses are no longer legally "invisible." The captain of the ship doctrine that protected them for so long from legal responsi-bility has been rightfully litigated out of existence in cases all across the country.[60-62]

The child abuse regulations require that those who are in a position to be aware of or suspect treatment that is defined as child abuse must report their concerns to child protective services. As the caregiver who has the closest and most enduring contact with infants, the nurse would certainly seem to bear a large measure of responsibility for monitoring the care of these vulnerable infants and acting on their behalf when necessary. Such actions might include explicit consultation with the neonatology staff to discuss alternative treatment, direct discussions of treatment options with parents, or referral of the case to the infant care review committee.

In spite of their special caregiver role with infants in the neonatal unit, however, primary care nurses are frequently excluded from the formal decision making process regarding withdrawal of treatment from handicapped newborns. There are various constraints, both internal and external, that may preclude nurses from taking a more active part in that process. For example, physician colleagues may underestimate the depth and breadth of nurses' knowledges about specific infants or undervalue their legitimacy as decision-makers. Nurses, themselves, may be hesitant or unwilling to become involved because they do not envision their role as one of decision-maker or because they are concerned about confronting the physician regarding treatment. Other variables such as poor communication among nurse and physician staff and infants' families or lack of effective mechanisms for review of cases such as case conferences or ethics committees may prevent or reduce nurse involvement in the decision making process.

The barriers to nurses' effective participation in the dialog and decision-making in these hard cases need to be eliminated. They can bring an invaluable perspective about the infant and his or her parents to the decision-making process. They often have close, frequent contact with families and provide information and strong support for the families as they are trying to make decisions about the infants' care. The nurses also try to help parents attach or bond to their infants over time, a critical variable that may shape parental decisions about the infant. Nurses' involvement in the decision-making process may help to ensure that just and humane decisions are made.

Summary

The unique nature of the nurse–infant relationship creates an ethical-legal obligation for neonatal nurses to advocate for treatment that is in the best interest of the handicapped infant. Nurses ought to play a pivotal role in helping to develop humane and just guidelines for the care of severely handicapped newborns by serving on infant care review committees, by interacting closely with state child protective services as they develop policies, and by working through professional associations to inform the courts as they evolve judicial rulings. Whether it is by design or default, the failure of nurses to become more actively involved in resolving treatment dilemmas does violence to their ethical code and to their covenant with infant patients.

References

[1] John A. Robertson (1983) *The Rights of the Critically Ill,* Bantam, New York, 88.

[2] *Federal Register* **49**: 238 (Dec. 10,1984) 48160–48169.

[3] President's Commission for the Study of Ethical Problems in Medicine and Biomedical and Behavioral Research (1983) *Deciding to Forego Life-Sustaining Treatment.* Washington, DC, 200–202.

[4] In re Quinlan, 70 NJ 10, 355 A 2d 647 (1976).

[5] Eichner v Dillon, 52 NY 2d 363 (1981).

[6] George J. Annas (1984) When Suicide Prevention Becomes Brutality: The Case of Elizabeth Bouvia. *The Hastings Center Report* **14**(3), 20–21, 46.

[7] Jeff Lyon (1985) *Playing God in the Nursery* W. W. Norton, New York.

[8] Joseph Fletcher (1972) Indicators of Humanhood: A Tentative Profile of Man, *The Hastings Center Report.*

[9] Michail Tooley (1979) Decisions to Terminate Life and the Concept of Person, in (John Ladd, ed.) *Ethical Issues Relating to Life and Death* , Cambridge.

[10] Roe v. Wade, 410 US 113 (1973).

[11] Robert A. McCormick (1974) To Save or Let Die— The Dilemma of Modern Medicine *Journal of the American Medical Association* **229**: 2, 174

[12] Paul Ramsey (1980) *Ethics at the Edge of Life,* Yale University Press, New Haven, 226.

[13] T.S. Powell, J.M. Aiken, and M.A. Smylie (1982) Treatment or Involuntary Euthanasia for Severely Handicapped Newborns: Issues of Philosophy and Public Policy. *The Association for Persons with Severe Handicaps Journal* **6**, 3–10.

[14] H. Rutherfor Turnbull, III (1986) Incidence of Infanticide in America: Public and Professional Attitudes. *Issues in Law and Medicine* **1**(5), 363–389.

[15] C. Everett Koop (1984) in *Selective Non-Treatment of Handicapped Newborns.*

[16]President's Commission, 217.

[17]Norm Fost (1978) Proxy Consent for Seriously Ill Newborns, in *No Rush to Judgment: Essays on Medical Ethics* (David H. Smith, ed.) The Poynter Center, Bloomington, Indiana.

[18]Norm Fost (1982) Putting Hospitals on Notice *The Hastings Center Report* 12(4), 5–8.

[19]William G. Bartholome (1986) Responsibilities to the Imperiled Infant. *Second Opinion* 2, 32–39.

[20]William G. Bartholome (1986) Clinical Ethics and the NICU. Paper presented at a conference sponsored by Carle Medical Foundation, San Diege, CA.

[21]Robert Weir (1984) *Selective Nontreatment of Handicapped Newborns.* Oxford University Press, New York, 188–223.

[22]John Lorber (1974) Selective Treatment of Myelomeningocele: To Treat or Not To Treat. *Pediatrics* 53, 307.

[23]John Freeman (1972) Is There a Right To Die Quickly? *Journal of Pediatrics* 80, 904.

[24]David G. McLone (1986) The Diagnosis, Prognosis, and Outcome for the Handicapped Newborn: A Neonatal View. *Issues in Law and Medicine* 2, 1, 15–24.

[25]R. Shurtleff (1974) Myelodysplasia: Decision for Death or Disability *New England Journal of Medicine* 291, 1005.

[26]*Johnson v Gross* (W. D. Okla. 1987) *See* alsoVictor G. Rosenblum and Edward R. Grant (1986) The Legal Response to Babies Doe: An Analytical Prognosis. *Issues in Law and Medicine,* 1(5), 401.

[27]Jehovah's Witness v. King County Hospital, 390 US 598 (1968).

[28]Custody of a Minor, 374 Mass. 733, 379 N.E. 2d 1053 (1978), aff'd 378 Mass. 732, 393 N.E. 2d 836 (1979).

[29]In re Cicero, 101 Misc. 2d 699 421 N.Y.S. 2d 965 (Sup. Ct. 1979).

[30]Guardianship of Philip B., 139 Cal. App. 3d 407, 188 Cal. Reptr., 781 (1983).

[31]Willard Gaylin and Ruth Macklin (eds) (1982) *Who Speaks for the Child,* Plenum, New York.

[32]John Robertson (1981) Dilemma in Danville. *The Hastings Center Report* 11(5), 5–7.

[33]James N. Gustafson (1973) Mongolism, Parental Desires, and the Right to Life. *Perspectives in Biology and Medicine* 16(4), 529–530.

[34]David H. Smith (1974) On Letting Some Babies Die. *Hastings Center Report* 2, 40–42.

[35]Who Shall Survive. (1972) Joseph P. Kennedy, Jr. Foundation, Washington DC.

[36]Raymond S. Duff and A.G. Campbell (1973) Moral and Ethical Dilemmas in the Special Care Nursery. *The New England Journal of Medicine* 289, 890–894.

[37]T.S. Ellis, III (1982) Letting Defective Babies Die: Who Decides? *American Journal of Law and Medicine* 7(4), 393–423.

[38]Diane Crane (1975) *The Sanctity of Human Life: Physicians' Treatment of Critically Ill Patients* Russell Sage Foundation, New York.

[39]Anthony Shaw, Judson G. Randolph, and Barbara Manard (1977) Ethical Issues in Pediatric Surgery: A National Survey of Pediatricians and Pediatric Surgeons. *Pediatrics* **60**, 588–599.

[40]David Todres (1977) Pediatricians' Attitudes Affecting Decision- Making In Defective Newborns. *Pediatrics* **60**, 197–201.

[41]John A. Robertson (1981) Dilemma in Danville. *The Hastings Center Report*, **11**(5) 5–7.

[42]Norm Fost, N. (1982) Putting Hospitals on Notice. *The Hastings Center Report*, **12**(2) 5–8.

[43]Ibid.

[44]Ibid.

[45]American Academy of Pediatrics v Heckler, No. 83-0774, US District Court, Washington, DC (April 14, 1983).

[46]Jeff Lyon (1985) *Playing God in the Nursery* p. 45–49.

[47]Weber v Stonybrook Hospital 467 NYS 2b 685 (1983).

[48]Weber v Stonybrook Hospital 465 NE 2d 1186 (1983).

[49]US v Univ. Hospital, 729 F. 2d 144 (2d Cir. 1984).

[50]Bowen v American Hospital Assoc. 106 S. Ct. 2101 (1986)

[51]David G. Mclone (1986) The Diagnosis, Prognosis, and Outcome for the Handicapped Newborn: A Neonatal View. *Issues in Law and Medicine*, **2**, 15–24.

[52]Federal Register 49:238 (December 10, 1984) p. 48160–48169.

[53]Federal Register 50:878 (April 15, 1985).

[54]Ibid.

[55]President's Commission for the Study of Ethical Principles in Medicine and Biomedical and Behavioral Research (1983) *Foregoing Life-Sustaining Treatment*, 197–229.

[56]Ibid., 218.

[57]Anne J. Davis and Mila A. Aroskar. (1983) *Ethical Dilemmas and Nursing Practice*. Appleton-Century-Crofts, Norwalk, Connecticut, p. 50.

[58]Ibid., 49.

[59]Sally Gadow (1980) Existential Advocacy: Philosophical Foundation of Nursing, in *Nurses: Images and Ideals*. Springer, New York, pp. 79–101.

[60]Goff v. Doctors General Hospital of San Jose, 166 Cal. App. 2d 314, 333 p. 2d 29 (1958).

[61]Sparger v. Worley Hospital, Inc. 547 S.W. 2d 582 (Tex, 1977).

[62]Adams v. Leidholdt, 579 p. 2d 618 (Colo. Supreme Court, 1978).

Index

179